Reversing DIABETES

FOOD PLAN + 70 DELICIOUS RECIPES

Dr Alan Barclay

MURDOCH BOOKS

Foreword
by Professor Jennie Brand-Miller

In *Reversing Diabetes*, Dr Alan Barclay takes the latest science and translates it into an accessible and practical guide. It provides the best, most accurate and up-to-date information on what you need to eat and do to successfully manage your diabetes – or even put it into remission – and if you have pre-diabetes, to turn back the clock.

Diabetes is a very complex condition and what works well for one person may not work for another. That's one reason why so many people with diabetes find that despite doing all the right things, their blood glucose levels fluctuate excessively and/or remain too high. The 70 recipes in this book provide options for people who choose to follow either lower carbohydrate or higher carbohydrate diets to manage their blood glucose levels. They come with a full nutritional analysis plus an estimated glycaemic index and glycaemic load value. Importantly, they are all suitable for people using a variety of different carbohydrate counting techniques to manage their diabetes including grams, exchanges or portions.

I am particularly delighted to write a foreword for this book, as its publication coincides with the twentieth anniversary of the publication of *The GI Factor* (now the *Low GI Diet Handbook*), which my colleagues and I wrote. We wanted to share the then ground-breaking findings that showed how simply swapping healthy low-GI foods and drinks for regular high-GI varieties within the same food group or category made an enormous difference to the diet and lifestyle of people with diabetes, giving some, in our experience, a new lease of life. Clinical trials have now clearly shown that using this GI approach, you can decrease your HbA1c by an average of 0.5 percentage points above and beyond what you would achieve by following a healthy diet alone. In addition, it may also decrease your risk of having a hypo (if you use insulin or other insulin-raising medications).

I recommend *Reversing Diabetes* with its practical information and delicious recipes that the whole family will enjoy as well as anyone with diabetes or pre-diabetes. It's also worth keeping in mind that a diet that's good for people with diabetes is a diet that's good for everybody.

Professor Jennie Brand-Miller, PhD, AM
Author of the *Low GI Diet* series and Professor of Human Nutrition,
Charles Perkins Centre, University of Sydney, Australia

R*eversing*
DIABETES

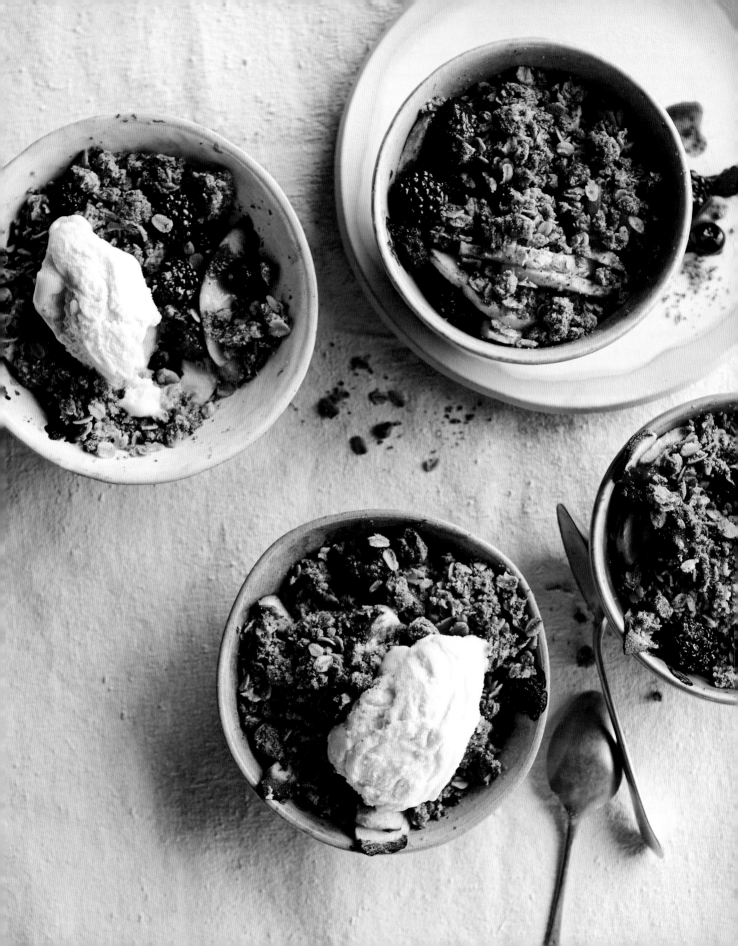

Foreword
by Professor Peter Colman

Diabetes, which affects at least 1.1 million Australians and costs the country $14 billion annually, provides major challenges for people living with the condition, their families, caring health professionals, the community and politicians. These challenges include reducing the prevalence of diabetes, detecting diabetes earlier in those at risk and reducing the complications that can occur if diabetes is not controlled optimally. Lifestyle approaches, in particular those addressing nutrition and physical exercise, are the common foundations in tackling the diabetes epidemic.

Reversing Diabetes will become a major resource in assisting people with diabetes or at high risk of developing diabetes. Alan Barclay's extremely broad experience in dietetics and diabetes science, research and clinical care place him in a unique position to 'put all the pieces together' for people trying to understand the way forward for their diabetes management.

There is up-to-date information on the causes of diabetes, the complications and most importantly the treatments and approaches to the prevention of diabetes. This is a rapidly developing field and the book captures the most recent developments. Of course, nutrition is key to all these domains and this is the area in which the book makes its biggest contribution. There is detailed and extremely thorough information guiding people through the many food choices available to them, allowing detailed analysis of the food groups for those requiring this level of detail. Sample meal plans are an added bonus for people wanting extra guidance.

I'm sure all diabetes health professionals will welcome Dr Barclay's excellent work and have no hesitation in recommending it as an essential reference for people with diabetes and their families.

Professor Peter Colman
Director, Department of Diabetes and Endocrinology,
Royal Melbourne Hospital

Preface

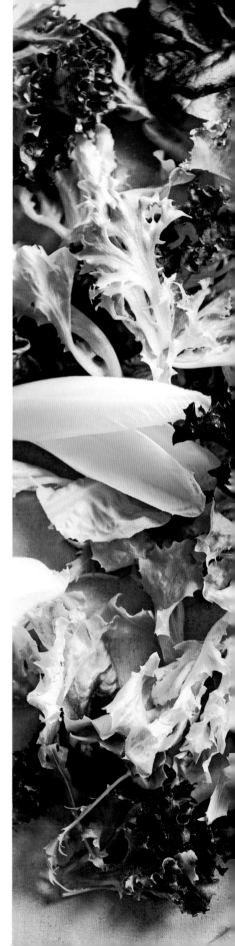

Diabetes has become a global pandemic. Consequently, preventing and even curing diabetes has become a major priority for governments and researchers alike. Each year, billions of dollars are spent around the globe on scientific research. Much of this research is published in journals or presented at conferences, and it's up to those working in the area of diabetes management and prevention to sift through the ever-expanding body of evidence to make sense of it all, to help guide future research and to advise people with existing diabetes and those at risk about the best way to prevent and manage the condition.

Regardless of what type of diabetes you have, chances are you have been advised that diabetes is a lifelong condition and that there is no cure. However, there is increasing evidence that you can at the very least delay the development of type 2 diabetes. Even if you do end up developing type 2 diabetes, if you treat it aggressively soon after you are diagnosed, you may be able to put it into remission using a variety of medical and non-medical treatments.

This is why we named this book *Reversing Diabetes* — to inspire you to explore these opportunities and see if you can indeed put your diabetes into remission. If you have type 1 diabetes, there is no convincing evidence at this point that you can reverse the condition through changes to your lifestyle, but you can delay or even prevent the development of the common complications of diabetes, and one of the simple ways you can do this is to ensure that you enjoy a healthy lifestyle that includes, of course, foods and drinks.

Drawing on over 20 years of clinical experience as an Accredited Practising Dietitian, including nearly 16 years at Diabetes Australia, I have combined the most recent and highest-quality evidence about the nutritional management and prevention of diabetes into one easy-to-read book that is jam-packed with practical everyday advice and 70 delicious

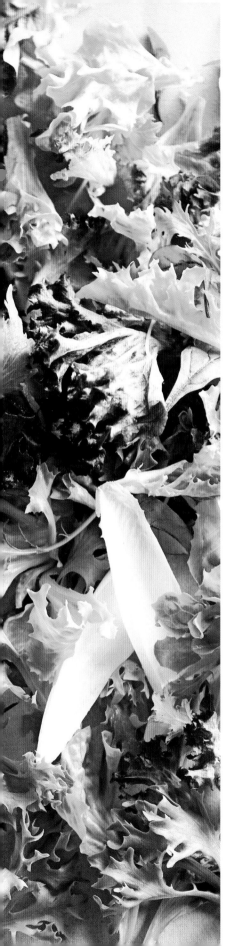

recipes. It will help you put the latest science into practice so that you can enjoy your food, while looking after your health as best as scientifically possible.

Food is much more than a collection of nutrients: it provides pleasure and is an important component of our culture as well as an expression of our individuality. It is important that people with diabetes, or those at risk, maintain the pleasure of eating by only limiting food choices when indicated by the best available scientific evidence.

While specifically designed for people with diabetes and those at risk, *Reversing Diabetes* is suitable for everyone who is interested in enjoying a healthy lifestyle. It covers topical issues that will not only help you to maintain your blood glucose levels as best as possible, but also your blood pressure, blood fats and body weight. It is suitable for people who are using a variety of different carbohydrate counting techniques including grams, exchanges and portions. It contains glycaemic index (GI) and glycaemic load (GL) estimates and full nutrition information, including gluten-free information, so that you can make fully informed decisions about what dishes best suit your individual needs. The book includes 70 recipes for everyday and special occasion cooking, from a broad range of cuisines, to maximise your enjoyment of food, and it includes recipes for different household sizes, including a range of recipes for two. It provides options for people who are following either a lower carbohydrate diet (for example Mediterranean) or a higher carbohydrate diet (for example Asian), to meet both your health and cultural needs.

Enjoy!

Dr Alan Barclay, PhD

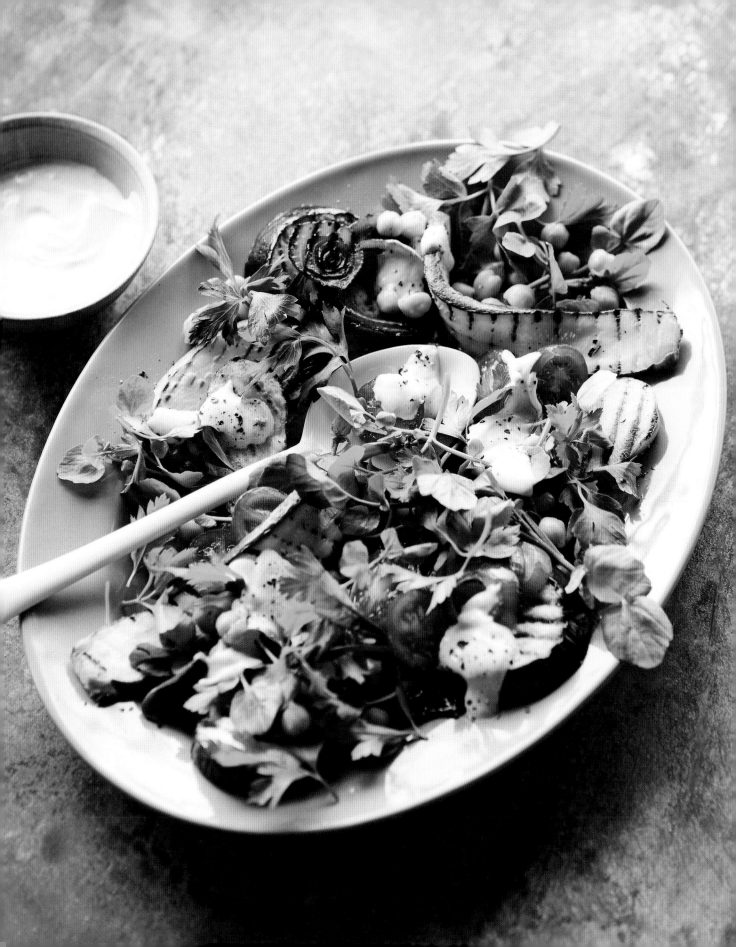

Contents

Part One
THE SCIENCE OF DIABETES AND PRE-DIABETES

Chapter One
UNDERSTANDING DIABETES AND PRE-DIABETES

DIABETES IS A DISEASE THAT DEVELOPS WHEN the body either stops producing the hormone insulin or when the insulin that it produces is not working properly. It has been around for many thousands of years, but was relatively uncommon until the last few decades of the twentieth century. It is now reaching what some people consider to be global pandemic proportions. The International Diabetes Federation estimates show that just under one in 10 adults, or 382 million people, have diabetes. This is expected to rise to 592 million people by the year 2035.

Diabetes is a Greek word that means to 'siphon' or 'pass through', which refers to the passing of liquid through the body, or frequent urination — one of the key symptoms of diabetes. The other classic signs of developing diabetes are increased hunger and thirst. These symptoms are caused by higher than normal blood glucose levels.

Glucose is a form of sugar and an essential fuel for most of the body's organs. Insulin acts like a key to open the doors to the cells to let in glucose from the blood. The glucose is used in the cells for fuel and to perform all different kinds of work. When blood glucose levels get too high, the kidneys flush the excess glucose out of the body. This can make you very thirsty and, because you are losing energy (in the form of glucose), hungry.

Types of diabetes

There are three main types of diabetes: type 1, type 2 and gestational. Whatever type of diabetes you have, one of the foundations of successful management is healthy eating and drinking. While there are a few differences between the way the different types are managed, the basic principles are much the same.

TYPE 1 DIABETES

In type 1 diabetes, the pancreas no longer produces insulin. While the exact reason for this is unknown, it is thought that the body's immune system is tricked into attacking and destroying most, if not all, of the insulin-producing beta cells in the pancreas. People with type 1 diabetes must take some form of insulin every day by either injection or a pump.

Around 10 in 100 people with diabetes have the type 1 form. It occurs most commonly in childhood and adolescence, but can also develop later in life.

TYPE 2 DIABETES

In type 2 diabetes, the pancreas is able to produce insulin, but either it does not produce enough to meet all of the body's requirements or the body's cells no longer respond to its effects due to insulin resistance. The exact cause of type 2 diabetes is also unknown and it is likely that there are different causes for different people.

Initially, people with type 2 diabetes can often manage their condition with a healthy diet and an increase in physical activity. However, as time passes, the majority end up requiring oral medications, and some people even end up having to use insulin.

Some risk factors for type 2 diabetes that can be influenced by lifestyle are: being overweight or obese (especially around the abdomen), having a poor diet and being physically inactive. Risk factors that we are unable to change include: our family history, ethnic background and advancing age.

GESTATIONAL DIABETES

Pregnant women who develop insulin resistance and subsequent elevated blood glucose levels are

Insulin resistance

Insulin resistance means that the insulin the pancreas is producing is not working as effectively as it should. It's a bit like a jammed door — more pressure is needed to open it. The pancreas then needs to produce more insulin to move glucose (and other nutrients) from the blood into the muscles, organs and tissues so they can function normally.

women who are over the age of 30, and women who are from certain ethnic backgrounds, such as Asian, Australian Aboriginal, Indian, Maori, Mediterranean and Pacific Islander.

Pre-diabetes

People with pre-diabetes (also known as 'impaired glucose tolerance' or 'impaired fasting glycaemia') have higher than normal blood glucose levels, but the levels are not high enough for a diagnosis of diabetes. In other words, people with pre-diabetes are in the grey area between having normal blood glucose levels and developing type 2 diabetes. If you have been diagnosed with pre-diabetes, think of it as an early warning, because it indicates that you are at high risk of developing type 2 diabetes.

There is strong evidence that losing a moderate amount of weight (around 7.5% of your body weight), improving your diet and increasing your physical activity levels can prevent pre-diabetes developing into type 2 diabetes. Nearly six out of 10 people can stop this from happening by taking these preventative steps.

said to have gestational diabetes. It usually occurs around the twenty-fourth week of pregnancy. Once the baby has been born, gestational diabetes usually goes away, but it is a sign that you are at increased risk of developing type 2 diabetes later in life.

Women with gestational diabetes are typically able to manage their condition with a healthy diet and some moderate exercise. However, insulin or oral medications are required in some cases.

Around one in 20 women develop gestational diabetes during pregnancy. It is more common in

Diabetes complications

There have been rapid developments in diabetes medications, blood glucose monitoring technology and our understanding of lifestyle management over the past few decades. These factors have all helped dramatically increase the average life expectancy and quality of life of people with diabetes. Despite this, there are a number of complications that can develop if the condition is not diagnosed early and effectively managed, which ultimately may reduce life expectancy.

The most common complications that occur in people with diabetes include:
- retinopathy, which affects the eyes
- neuropathy and peripheral vascular disease, which affect the feet
- kidney disease (nephropathy)
- erectile dysfunction, which causes impotence
- cardiovascular disease, which affects the heart and blood vessels in the brain
- periodontal disease, which affects the gums.

The good news is that it is possible to prevent, or at the very least delay, the development of these complications through the optimal management of the condition.

Why is type 2 diabetes rapidly increasing around the globe?

There are many reasons why type 2 diabetes rates are increasing, but it's not all bad news.

AGEING POPULATION

The older you are, the greater your risk of developing type 2 diabetes because your pancreas, along with other vital organs, wears out with advancing age. Also, the slow but steady weight gain that occurs over the course of a lifetime slowly increases insulin resistance. So, perhaps surprisingly, increasing diabetes rates are a sign of our recent success as a species in increasing life expectancy.

PHYSICAL INACTIVITY

Increasing mechanisation of the home, the workplace and transport has dramatically decreased the average level of physical activity in both the developed and developing world over the last few decades. This trend has helped liberate many people from tedious, back-breaking work, and helped provide us with more leisure time. However, it has also led to a decrease in muscle mass, an increase in body fat and associated insulin resistance, increasing the risk of developing type 2 and gestational diabetes.

FOOD AND NUTRITION

Around the globe, increased participation of both men and women in the workforce has led to an increased reliance on processed, pre-prepared meals and foods that are eaten away from home. While these meals and foods are undoubtedly convenient and tasty, many are based on highly refined ingredients and they are often energy dense, but nutrient poor.

REVERSING DIABETES

DIABETES IS A LIFELONG CONDITION AND THERE is, as yet, no cure. One of the reasons why we haven't found a cure is that all types of diabetes are extremely complicated, and we don't yet fully understand what causes them. However, billions of dollars are spent around the globe each year in trying to find out more about how our bodies work, what goes wrong when we develop diabetes, and how we can prevent, delay or cure it. While we haven't yet found a cure, we know how we can prevent or at least delay the development of type 2 diabetes, and even reverse it in some people. Trials are also underway that may help prevent type 1 diabetes in some people in the not-too-distant future.

Clinical trials into preventing type 2 diabetes

Over the last couple of decades, clinical trials have been conducted around the world to see if people with pre-diabetes can prevent or at least delay the development of type 2 diabetes. As well as returning blood glucose levels to the normal range, one of the primary goals of the trials has been to modestly reduce body weight — by between 5 and 10% of a person's weight.

The weight loss was typically achieved through a moderate reduction in kilojoules (around 2000 kJ less each day) as part of an overall healthy eating plan. The plan was reduced in fat (25 to 30% of kilojoules), low in saturated fat (7 to 10% of kilojoules) and high in dietary fibre (at least 3.5 g for every 1000 kJ consumed). Participants were also advised to do at least 150 minutes of moderate intensity activity each week (e.g. five 30-minute sessions of brisk walking) to assist with their weight loss and to decrease their insulin resistance.

A review of all the diabetes prevention trials that have been conducted so far was recently published, incorporating over 8000 people from around the world. The review found that lifestyle interventions could decrease the risk of people with pre-diabetes from developing type 2 diabetes by over 50%, which is a huge reduction.

In addition, there is very strong evidence from observational studies that healthy, low-glycaemic index (GI) and low-glycaemic load (GL) diets may decrease the risk of developing diabetes by up to 45%. Observational studies are studies measuring the lifestyle habits of large groups of healthy people for 5 to 20+ years. Because these kinds of studies do not prove cause and effect, research is currently underway that will help conclusively prove whether or not low-GI and low-GL diets can prevent the development of type 2 diabetes.

There is strong evidence from observational studies that healthy low-glycaemic index and low-glycaemic load diets may decrease the risk of developing diabetes by up to 45%.

Can type 2 diabetes be reversed?

While type 2 diabetes cannot be cured as such, it can be put in to remission in people who have been newly diagnosed if they are able to lose a significant amount of body weight and keep it off. We use the word 'remission' rather than 'cure' because diabetes may return years later, either due to people slowly regaining weight or simply due to advancing age.

There are three approaches that are used to try to fight diabetes when it is newly diagnosed: weight loss through lifestyle changes, weight loss through bariatric (weight loss) surgery and the use of insulin.

LIFESTYLE CHANGES

Clinical trials show that around one in eight people can put type 2 diabetes into remission for between 2 and 10 years by losing a significant amount of body weight as a result of following a healthy lifestyle.

BARIATRIC SURGERY

Bariatric surgery is a radical treatment that can also put type 2 diabetes into remission. It includes a variety of surgical procedures performed on people who are obese, and includes reducing the size of the stomach with a gastric band or removal of a portion to form a small stomach pouch, or by re-routing the small bowel to a small stomach pouch. In the medium to long term (2 to 5 years), it is more effective than lifestyle interventions, helping between three and seven out of 10 people to go into remission.

If you are considering bariatric surgery, consult your doctor, who will work with you to weigh up the risks and benefits, and the financial costs. There is a range of possible side effects of bariatric surgery, some of which can be life-threatening, so the decision needs to be made very carefully.

SHORT-TERM INSULIN USE

A review of clinical trials has shown that short-term (2 to 3 weeks) use of insulin by those newly diagnosed with type 2 diabetes can cause medium-term (2 years) remission in about four out of 10 people.

It is up to your doctor and you to decide what, if any, medicines to utilise when you are first diagnosed. While some people are afraid of injecting themselves with insulin, modern needles are relatively fine, and most people think the injections are less painful than pricking your finger for blood glucose monitoring.

Preventing gestational diabetes

Women who have had gestational diabetes are at a significantly increased risk of developing it again with subsequent pregnancies, and of developing type 2 diabetes later in life. Advice for preventing type 2 diabetes is relevant to women who have previously had gestational diabetes and want to prevent it from happening again.

Managing gestational diabetes

Because pregnancy lasts around 9 months, and gestational diabetes is typically diagnosed around 6 months, it cannot be reversed as such. However, gestational diabetes can be managed through a careful combination of healthy eating and moderate, regular physical activity, and in some cases insulin or medication.

Once the baby is born, gestational diabetes usually goes away. If you have another baby, you are at greater risk of developing gestational diabetes. Advice for preventing type 2 diabetes is relevant to women who want to avoid developing gestational diabetes again.

Can type 1 diabetes be prevented?

Until recently, most health professionals would have agreed that type 1 diabetes cannot be prevented. However, current research shows that the increasing rates of type 1 diabetes that have been seen in recent years in Australia and the UK may be due to an increase in the number of children and adolescents who are more sensitive to environmental factors, rather than genetic factors. This means that the potential role of lifestyle in the development of type 1 diabetes needs to be carefully considered.

One of these environmental factors is growing rates of insulin resistance at an earlier age due to our increasing rates of overweight and obesity, and increasingly sedentary lifestyles. There are also some potential environmental triggers such as diets low in omega-3 fats and vitamin D, or diets with a high GI, certain infant feeding practices, or factors that affect an individual's microbiome. It is important to note that these lifestyle factors are yet to be proven risk factors, and that other factors such as bacterial and viral infections are equally likely triggers of type 1 diabetes that are also being investigated.

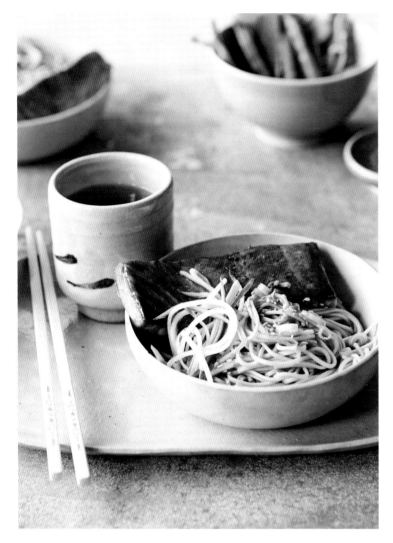

Teriyaki salmon with soba noodles and pickled vegetables is a good source of omega-3 fats.
Recipe page 126

muscle mass, which in turn gobbles up blood glucose as its preferred fuel. So increasing physical activity has more benefits than just helping to lose body fat, it can also help reduce the body's insulin requirements. This is an important part of the preventing-diabetes jigsaw puzzle.

OMEGA-3 FATS

Diets that are high in omega-3 fats (found primarily in fatty fish like salmon, herring, sardines, mackerel and anchovies) are associated with decreased risk of type 1 diabetes in a growing number of observational studies. It is thought that these fats may decrease the body's inflammatory response, reducing the damage to the beta (insulin-producing) cells that are found in the pancreas.

VITAMIN D

Several studies from around the world have found an increase in the risk of developing type 1 diabetes in children with low vitamin D levels. It is thought that adequate vitamin D levels help to regulate the body's immune system, decreasing its tendency to attack the insulin-producing beta cells.

INSULIN RESISTANCE AND INFLAMMATION

Carrying excess body fat, especially around the abdomen, is one of the factors that has been linked to insulin resistance. It is also thought to increase the production of a range of inflammatory hormones that may increase the risk of autoimmune diseases like type 1 diabetes.

Physical activity increases insulin sensitivity — the flip side of insulin resistance — by increasing lean

Given the amount of sunshine in Australia, it is hard to believe that around 10% of Australians are deficient in vitamin D. Perhaps less surprising is the fact that around 16% of people living in the UK are deficient in vitamin D. All most people need is 15 to 30 minutes of upper body (face, neck and arms) sun exposure, two to three times a week. This is not hard to achieve living in most parts of Australia, but it is more of a challenge in the UK. Unfortunately, few foods contain significant amounts of vitamin D. Fortified margarine is the major dietary source, along with fatty fish such as salmon, herring and mackerel, and eggs.

HIGH-GLYCAEMIC INDEX (GI) DIETS

While the evidence linking high-GI diets to the risk of developing type 2 diabetes is compelling, no one had investigated the connection of high-GI diets to the development of type 1 diabetes until recently. One study looked at the diet of nearly 2000 American children who were at risk of developing type 1 diabetes. It found that a high-GI diet increases the risk of type 1 diabetes in children who have already developed antibodies to the beta cells in their pancreas. This is because the high-GI diet may be increasing insulin resistance, adding to the stress put on the remaining beta cells and hastening the development of type 1 diabetes in already susceptible young people.

Antibodies

An antibody is a kind of protein produced by white blood cells that is used by our immune systems to identify and neutralise pathogens like bacteria and viruses. For some as yet unknown reason, people with type 1 diabetes have developed antibodies to the beta cells that are contained within islets in the pancreas. Over time, this leads to the development of the condition.

INFANT FEEDING

There is growing evidence that some children who are fed infant formulas based on cow's milk are at increased risk of developing type 1 diabetes compared to those who are breastfed. There are two main theories for this increased risk.

1) An infant's developing body may develop an immune reaction ('allergy') to certain proteins found in cow's milk formulas that are similar to those found in the insulin-producing cells in the pancreas, attacking and eventually destroying them over time.

2) Susceptible infants may miss out on immune factors found in their mother's milk or obtained from their mother's breast tissue (for example, beneficial bacteria) if they are not breastfed.

What is our microbiome?

Our microbiome is a collection of around 100 trillion bacteria (mostly), fungi and viruses that live on the surface of our bodies and inside our gastrointestinal tracts, or guts. A typical adult's microbiome weighs around 1 kilogram, equivalent to some of our essential organs. There are about 10 times more bacteria in our microbiome than there are cells in our body. In other words, 90% of the cells in our bodies are microbial and only the remaining 10% are human!

MICROBIOME

Some of the many factors that affect our microbiome include whether we had a normal birth or were born via caesarean section, whether we were breastfed or bottle fed, what foods we were weaned on to, and what we habitually eat. Diets that are high in plant fibres, fermented foods and drinks are thought to be beneficial, while highly processed, low-fibre foods full of preservatives may be harmful to our microbiome.

Small bowel (intestine) biopsies from children with type 1 diabetes have found that intestinal immune cells are activated in about half of the children and partly as a consequence the gut wall is also more permeable, potentially allowing small proteins and bacteria into the bloodstream. Because the pancreas is joined to the small intestine, any disturbances to the gut microbiome may lead to the development of type 1 diabetes in some people.

TIPS FOR THOSE AT RISK OF TYPE 1 DIABETES

While research that links lifestyle factors to the development of type 1 diabetes may provide hope to some parents who have children at increased risk, much more research is needed before we can make any strong recommendations. However, most of the dietary factors discussed here are not that difficult to adopt and may have health benefits for the whole family even if research eventually shows that they do not help prevent type 1 diabetes. For example:

- prevent children and adolescents from becoming either overweight or underweight
- help them to eat sufficient foods and drinks to grow and develop normally
- ensure regular physical activity is an important part of the whole family's life
- enjoy one or more serves of fatty fish like salmon, herring or sardines at least three times each week
- enjoy healthy high-fibre foods and limit highly processed and preserved foods
- enjoy fermented milk products like plain yoghurt.

Can type 1 diabetes be reversed?

At this stage, there is no evidence that type 1 diabetes can be reversed through lifestyle changes. Islet cell and whole pancreas transplants are available now for some people with type 1 diabetes, however. Extensive research is also underway, from stem cell transplants to closed loop insulin pumps, that may lead to a 'cure' for type 1 diabetes in the not-too-distant future.

UNDERSTANDING BLOOD GLUCOSE, BLOOD FATS AND BLOOD PRESSURE

HAVING THE HIGHER THAN IDEAL BLOOD GLUCOSE levels that are a symptom of diabetes can have severe consequences over many years, but many people with diabetes or pre-diabetes also have higher than normal blood cholesterol, triglycerides or blood pressure. This may also increase the risk of common complications. Like blood glucose levels, these risk factors can be improved through a combination of healthy eating, regular physical activity and appropriate medication.

Blood glucose

Because it is one of the body's preferred fuel sources, glucose levels in the blood are carefully maintained by insulin and glucagon, two powerful hormones that are produced in the pancreas. Insulin lowers blood glucose by allowing glucose into the body's cells. Glucagon raises blood glucose levels by causing the liver to release stored glucose into the bloodstream.

The brain and nervous system basically run on glucose for fuel. If they are to function normally, blood glucose levels need to be maintained between 3.5 and 6 mmol/L. If levels drop too low, you start to develop symptoms of hypoglycaemia (also known as a 'hypo') including sweating, trembling, confusion,

incoherent rambling speech, dizziness and lack of coordination (the order of symptoms can vary). If levels get too high, you experience increased thirst, urination and appetite. It can lead to ketoacidosis in the short term and increases the risk of cardiovascular disease and other complications in the long term.

MEASURING BLOOD GLUCOSE LEVELS

There are two main measures of blood glucose levels that are used to gauge how well people with diabetes are managing their condition. One measure looks at short-term blood glucose levels and the other looks at long-term blood glucose levels. Remember to use the information from both to optimise your diabetes management.

You can measure short-term blood glucose levels at home using a blood glucose monitor. How often you measure your blood glucose at home will be determined by your doctor, diabetes specialist, diabetes educator or dietitian. The decision will depend on a range of factors, including what type of diabetes you have, how you manage it and how often and intensely you exercise.

Blood glucose monitoring can inform the management of diabetes and therefore reduce the risk of complications. People with type 1 diabetes need to monitor their blood glucose at least four times a day. This is usually done before each main meal as well as before going to bed. People with type 2 diabetes who use insulin or medications that increase insulin production also need to monitor their blood glucose levels daily, but usually not as frequently as people who have type 1 diabetes.

Table 1: Recommended ranges for blood glucose, blood fats and blood pressure

HEALTH MEASURE	RECOMMENDED RANGE
Blood glucose levels	6–8 mmol/L fasting* 8–10 mmol/L after a meal or snack*
Glycosylated haemoglobin (HbA1c)	Less than or equal to 53 mmol/mol (range 48–58)* Less than or equal to 7% (range 6.5–7.5)*
Blood cholesterol	Total less than 4.0 mmol/L HDL greater than or equal to 1.0 mmol/L LDL less than 2.0 mmol/L
Blood triglycerides	Less than 2.0 mmol/L
Blood pressure	Less than or equal to 130/80 mmHg

Primarily for people with type 2 diabetes or pre-diabetes. People with type 1 diabetes may have different targets that should be determined in conjunction with their health professional team.

Source: General practice management of type 2 diabetes – 2014–15. RACGP and Diabetes Australia, 2014.

People with pre-diabetes, or type 2 diabetes managed through lifestyle or medications that do not increase insulin production don't need to routinely monitor their blood glucose using this method. However, it can be a useful tool to determine blood glucose patterns when first diagnosed and as a part of an annual blood glucose monitoring plan. Table 1 (above) lists the typical recommended ranges for blood glucose levels.

GLYCOSYLATED HAEMOGLOBIN

The most common long-term measure of blood glucose is known as glycosylated haemoglobin, or HbA1c for short. This chemical compound develops in the blood when haemoglobin (the protein in red blood cells that carries oxygen around the body) attaches to glucose in the blood, becoming glycosylated. The amount of glycated haemoglobin in your blood provides an overall picture of your

Ketoacidosis

Most cases of ketoacidosis occur in people with type 1 diabetes. It very rarely occurs in people with type 2 diabetes. Ketoacidosis is a serious health condition associated with acute illness, such as an infection, or very high blood glucose levels. It develops gradually over hours or days, and is a sign of insufficient insulin. Without enough insulin, the body's cells cannot use glucose for energy, so they switch over to burning fat. This leads to an accumulation of dangerous chemical substances in the blood called ketones, which also appear in the urine. Measure your urine or blood ketone levels and see your doctor if you experience any of the symptoms listed.

Symptoms

High blood glucose levels and ketones (in the urine or blood) with:
- rapid breathing
- flushed cheeks
- abdominal pain
- a sweet acetone smell (similar to nail polish remover) on the breath
- vomiting
- dehydration.

average blood glucose levels over a period of around 3 months. Research has shown that the higher the HbA1c level, the greater the risk of developing diabetes-related complications. HbA1c levels should be monitored every 3 to 6 months, and can be organised by your doctor as part of your diabetes management plan.

Clinical trials have found that people with diabetes who follow healthy eating principles can reduce their HbA1c levels by 1 to 2 percentage points. If they are also following a low-GI diet, their HbA1c levels can be reduced by another 0.5 percentage points. While this may not sound significant, a decrease of just 1 percentage point in HbA1c levels will decrease the common complications of diabetes by 16 to 43%.

Blood cholesterol and triglycerides (blood fats)

High levels of blood cholesterol and triglycerides are linked to the common complications of diabetes and also to each other.

CHOLESTEROL

Cholesterol is a fat that is a part of all of the body's cells. It is essential for many metabolic processes, including the production of hormones, vitamin D and bile for digesting fat, and absorbing fat-soluble vitamins from foods. It is produced primarily by the liver and also made by most cells in the body.

High triglyceride levels can be caused by a number of factors, including being overweight, a high-fat diet, too many high-GI carbohydrates, too much alcohol and not enough omega-3 fats.

Cholesterol is carried around in the blood by 'couriers' called lipoproteins, which include LDL or 'bad' cholesterol and HDL or 'good' cholesterol.

LDL, or low density lipoprotein cholesterol, carries cholesterol from the liver to the rest of the body's organs, where it can build up in the walls of blood vessels (arteries), eventually blocking them. Having high levels of LDL in the blood is therefore a risk factor for cardiovascular disease.

HDL, or high density lipoprotein cholesterol, seems to protect against cardiovascular disease because it clears cholesterol from the blood vessels and helps in its removal from the body. Having low levels of HDL in the blood is also a risk factor for cardiovascular disease.

TRIGLYCERIDES

Triglyceride is the scientific name for fat, and it can come from dietary fat, or it can be manufactured in the body from other nutrients. High blood triglyceride levels are a risk factor for cardiovascular disease in people with diabetes. Having too much triglyceride in the blood is often linked with having too little HDL cholesterol.

There are a number of factors that can cause high triglyceride levels, including being overweight, consuming a high-fat diet, eating too many highly refined carbohydrates, drinking too much alcohol and not eating enough omega-3 polyunsaturated fats (primarily from seafoods).

Optimal ranges for cholesterol and triglyceride levels are listed in Table 1 (see page 13).

Blood pressure

Blood pressure is simply the pressure of the blood against the walls of the blood vessels as it is pumped around the body by the heart. As the heart pumps and relaxes, blood pressure rises and falls in a regular wave-like pattern, so blood pressure peaks when your heart pumps (systolic blood pressure) and falls when your heart relaxes (diastolic blood pressure). High blood pressure is a risk factor for heart attack or stroke, so ask your doctor to monitor it regularly.

Key dietary factors that influence blood pressure include salt or sodium intake, potassium intake and calcium intake. Eating too many kilojoules, leading to weight gain, can increase blood pressure. Regular physical activity can help reduce blood pressure.

DIABETES MYTHS

MYTHS ABOUT DIABETES ARE PLENTIFUL AND prevalent, so much so that it would be possible to write a whole book on them. Below are some of the more popular myths that are currently circulating.

Myth 1: Sugar causes diabetes

This has to be the greatest of all myths about diabetes. Diabetes has been around for thousands of years, and we worked out long ago that it had something to do with excess sugar in the urine. Treatments varied from culture to culture and throughout time, but generally focused on either eating more sugars (to replace what was being lost in the urine) or restricting sugars (to reduce losses in the urine), with varying degrees of success. We now know that the sugar in the urine that is characteristic of diabetes is glucose. We also know that essentially all of the carbohydrate we eat, whether it is from starchy or sugary foods, ends up as glucose.

A recent review of the evidence from large observational studies looked at the intake of total carbohydrates, sugars (glucose, fructose, sucrose and lactose) and starch, and the risk of developing type 2 diabetes. The review found an overall lack of evidence of an association between any of them.

However, the evidence from large observational studies shows that diets that have a high average glycaemic index (GI) or glycaemic load (GL) are strongly associated with a risk of type 2 diabetes.

Observational studies also suggest that excessive consumption of sugar-sweetened beverages (more than one to two 355 ml drinks a day) is associated with an increased risk of developing type 2 diabetes. There is further evidence associating diet soft drinks with the risk of developing type 2 diabetes.

Unlike randomised controlled trials, observational studies do not prove causality and so more research is needed to determine if these suspected links are real. It could be, for example, that people who usually drink regular or diet soft drinks do so along with other highly processed foods, such as potato chips (crisps and fries), savoury snacks and pastries, or alcohol (scotch and cola, for example). If so, it is perhaps the overall dietary pattern of highly refined food consumption that's really to blame.

There is evidence from randomised controlled trials that the best way to reduce the risk of developing type 2 diabetes is to consume 2000 to 2500 less kilojoules each day by eating less fat, particularly reducing saturated fat and increasing dietary fibre. Many people can also reduce their kilojoule intake by reducing their consumption of added sugars.

The bottom line is that sugar itself does not cause diabetes.

Randomised controlled trials

Randomised controlled trials in humans are considered the 'gold standard' as they can prove that intervention A improves health outcome B, while all other known factors (known as confounders) have been accounted for by randomisation. For example, two groups of people are fed two different diets and their health status is measured over a period of a few weeks to several years. Having a control group is vital in order to enable you to compare the two different interventions.

Myth 2: People with diabetes should not have sugar

The world's major diabetes associations (American Diabetes Association, Canadian Diabetes Association, Diabetes Australia and Diabetes UK) are in agreement that sugar-free diets should not be recommended to people living with diabetes. The reasons for this are simple: sugars and starches (see page 31) are all digested, absorbed and metabolised to the sugar glucose. Therefore people with diabetes need to carefully balance the type and amounts of all carbohydrate that they eat and drink each day to ensure their blood glucose levels do not go too high or too low, not simply limit the amount of sugars.

As with most things in life, moderation is the key. People with diabetes, like everyone else, should consume added sugars in moderation — no more than 10% of total energy (less than 55 g) a day for the average adult.

Myth 3: Low-carbohydrate diets are best for people with diabetes

There is evidence that a range of different eating patterns can help people to manage their blood glucose levels in the short to medium term. People consuming low-carbohydrate, low-GI, Mediterranean, vegetarian and high-protein diets for at least 6 months will lower their HbA1c by 0.12 to 0.47 percentage points, with the low-carbohydrate diet providing the 0.12% reduction and the Mediterranean diet providing the 0.47% reduction.

For most people, diabetes is a lifelong condition, and food is one of life's great pleasures. It is therefore wise to choose an eating pattern that you enjoy, that also helps you manage your diabetes well and that you can live with the rest of your days, and not simply follow the latest dietary trend.

Current scientific evidence indicates that non-nutritive sweeteners are safe to consume in moderate amounts, and that they can be useful for reducing consumption of added nutritive sweeteners.

Myth 4: Non-nutritive sweeteners are worse than sugar

Non-nutritive or 'artificial' sweeteners have been around for over a century, helping people to enjoy sweet foods and drinks without the unwanted kilojoules or carbohydrate that can contribute to weight gain and raise blood glucose levels when consumed in excess. There is very strong evidence that non-nutritive sweeteners do not raise blood glucose levels in the short term, but there is some emerging evidence in animals that they may increase the risk of developing type 2 diabetes. Also, there has been conflicting evidence about the effect of these sweeteners on body weight.

ARTIFICIAL SWEETENERS AND THE RISK OF DIABETES

In late 2014, a study linking the artificial sweeteners aspartame, sucralose and saccharin to the risk of diabetes hit the headlines around the globe. The fact that most of this research was conducted in mice was lost in the reporting. The mice were overfed pure saccharin — the sweetener identified by the research as the most potent of the artificial sweeteners under investigation. The result was that it altered their glucose tolerance and gut bacteria (microbiome).

To put the research into context, saccharin was discovered in 1879 and the diabetes epidemic has only developed around the world over the last few decades. The use of saccharin is decreasing — it is no longer a particularly popular sweetener. Aspartame (which was included in the study, but found to be less potent), stevia and cyclamate are much more widely used. Finally, the rodents were fed around 17 times more saccharin than a typical adult consumes (according to the results of Australia's most recent sweetener survey).

The results of the research can be considered interesting at best, but they definitely don't provide convincing evidence that 'artificial' sweeteners cause diabetes as the headlines suggested. More research is definitely needed before we can draw that conclusion.

ARTIFICIAL SWEETENERS AND WEIGHT

Recent headlines have suggested that despite the fact that they are very low in kilojoules, using 'artificial' sweeteners may actually make you gain weight. A recent systematic review looked at all published randomised controlled trials and observational studies about body weight. This review found that the use of low- and no-calorie sweeteners led to small but statistically significant improvements in body weight, body mass index, fat mass and waist circumference in randomised controlled trials. In observational studies, however, the use of low- and no-calorie sweeteners was not associated with improvements in body weight or fat mass, but was in fact significantly associated with slightly higher body mass index. Overall, the evidence from the randomised controlled trials is more powerful than the evidence from the observational studies.

The bottom line is that current scientific evidence indicates that non-nutritive sweeteners are safe to consume in moderate amounts, and that they can be useful for reducing some people's consumption of added nutritive sweeteners, helping them to lose weight, provided they do not treat themselves with other highly processed foods and drinks as a reward for avoiding the added sugars.

Whenever you see sensationalist headlines claiming that a particular sweetener causes obesity, diabetes and so on, ask yourself if the research was conducted in humans, and whether you consume the amount of sweetener the participants were fed on a regular basis over a long period of time. If your answer is no, chances are that the research finding does not have any relevance for you. However, if you choose to use an alternative sweetener to help reduce your kilojoule intake or manage your blood glucose levels, do so in moderation (as in all things), and use a variety of non-nutritive sweeteners to reduce the likelihood of excessive consumption of any particular one.

DIABETES AND COELIAC DISEASE

COELIAC DISEASE IS BECOMING INCREASINGLY common, affecting around one in 100 people in the UK and Australia, and one in 133 Americans. For reasons that we do not yet completely understand, people with type 1 diabetes are at up to 10 times greater risk of developing coeliac disease than people who do not have type 1 diabetes.

Like type 1 diabetes, coeliac disease is thought to be an autoimmune disease that is 'triggered' in genetically susceptible people. Unfortunately, coeliac disease can make management of blood glucose levels even harder than usual in people with type 1 diabetes, with an increased risk of both hyperglycaemia and hypoglycaemia. People with type 2 diabetes or pre-diabetes are believed to have the same chance of having coeliac disease as the rest of the population.

The immune system of those with coeliac disease reacts abnormally to the protein gluten that is found in wheat, rye and barley (and is a common contaminant in oats), causing damage to the small bowel (intestine). The tiny, finger-like projections known as villi that line the small intestine become inflamed and flattened, a condition that is known as villous atrophy. As a consequence, the surface area of the intestine available for the absorption of nutrients is reduced, which can lead to various gastrointestinal and malabsorptive symptoms like diarrhoea; constipation; large, bulky, foul stools; unwanted weight loss or poor growth in children; flatulence; abdominal bloating, distension or pain; and anaemia. Long-term complications can be very serious and include infertility, miscarriage, depression and dental enamel defects. There is also an increased risk of developing certain forms of cancer such as lymphoma of the small bowel.

If you have a family history of coeliac disease, some or even all of these symptoms, it's important that you don't simply self-diagnose coeliac disease and commence a gluten-free diet. A diagnosis of coeliac disease can only be made by demonstrating the typical villous atrophy of coeliac disease in a small bowel biopsy. This involves a gastroscopy in which several tiny samples of the small bowel are taken and examined under a microscope. It is important that you are still eating gluten regularly before the procedure is performed or you may get a false negative result.

GLUTEN INTOLERANCE
Some people believe that they are sensitive to gluten, even though small bowel biopsy results show that they don't have coeliac disease. When

people with gluten intolerance avoid gluten, their gastrointestinal symptoms generally improve. However, a recent Australian study suggests that people with so-called gluten intolerance may not in fact be sensitive to gluten as such. Indeed, their gut symptoms may be due to other dietary factors, in particular, fermentable, poorly absorbed short-chain carbohydrates, that is fermentable, oligo-, di-, monosaccharides and polyols (FODMAPs) that are found in a wide range of foods. Rather than simply avoiding gluten, people with these symptoms may instead benefit from a low FODMAPs diet.

Because the symptoms of non-coeliac gluten sensitivity can be very similar to coeliac disease, or other conditions, it is important that you don't self-diagnose and go on a gluten-free diet — see your doctor first.

Gluten-free foods

Following a gluten-free diet is currently the only known treatment for coeliac disease. Unfortunately, the diet needs to be followed for life because those with coeliac disease remain sensitive to gluten their whole lives. At this point in time, the condition can't be cured as such. However, by removing the cause of the disease, a gluten-free diet allows the small bowel lining to heal and symptoms to resolve. As long as the gluten-free diet is strictly adhered to, the problems arising from coeliac disease should not return.

In the not-too-distant past, having to consume a gluten-free diet was a culinary disaster. Thankfully, there are now gluten-free alternatives available for most foods. Many gluten-free core foods like milk, yoghurt, some starchy vegetables, legumes and most fruits also have a low GI (glycaemic index. See page 34). However, many gluten-free grain alternatives aren't low GI, so finding suitable gluten-free breads, pasta and breakfast cereals can still be a challenge for those diagnosed with both coeliac disease and diabetes.

Unless you have diagnosed coeliac disease or require a low FODMAPs diet, you probably don't need to be avoiding gluten, and don't need to purchase gluten-free foods.

A selection of recipes within *Reversing Diabetes* are gluten free, as indicated in the recipe nutrition information panel.

Lower-GI gluten-free foods

Always carefully check the ingredients panel of packaged foods as different brands of the same product may contain gluten.

GRAINS
- Buckwheat
- Cellophane noodles
- Corn tortillas
- Some brown and white rice varieties labelled low GI
- Rice vermicelli
- Soba noodles
- Quinoa
- Wild rice

BREAKFAST CEREALS
- Buckwheat kernels
- Rice bran
- Some varieties of muesli

FRUIT
- Most fresh, frozen, dried, glacé or tinned fruits
- 100% fruit juices

VEGETABLES
- Butternut pumpkin (squash)
- Carisma potatoes
- Corn
- Taro
- Yam

LEGUMES
- Dried and tinned beans, peas, lentils or chickpeas

DAIRY AND SOY
- Low-fat ice cream
- Low-fat and reduced-fat milk
- Low-fat and reduced-fat soy drinks (calcium fortified)
- Yoghurt

SNACK FOODS
- Plain popcorn
- Nuts
- Dried fruit and nut mixes
- Sunflower seeds and pepitas (pumpkin seeds)

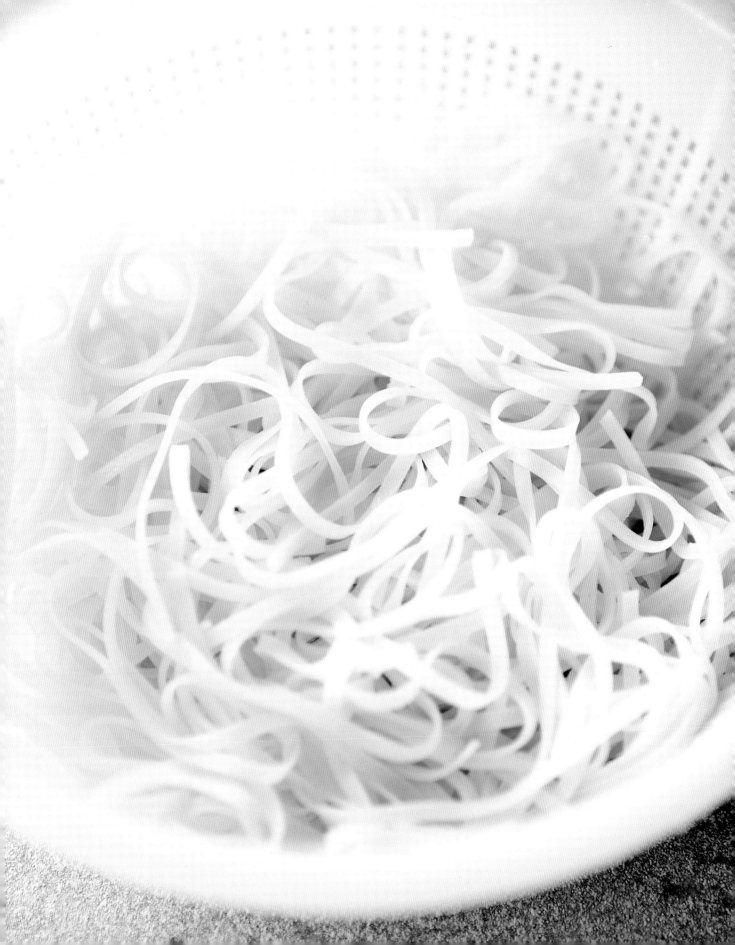

Chapter Two
HEALTHY EATING WITH DIABETES AND PRE-DIABETES

BEFORE DELVING MORE DEEPLY INTO THE FOOD and nutrition recommendations for people with diabetes or those at risk, it's important to think about the broader goals that we are all trying to achieve.

When you have a chronic condition like diabetes that is profoundly affected by the foods and drinks you consume, there can be a tendency to focus more on the health aspects of food and nutrition, and to focus less on the enjoyment of eating. This is a shame, because food is much more than a collection of nutrients: it is one of life's greatest pleasures and is an important component of our culture, as well as an expression of our individuality. We use certain foods and drinks to celebrate all of the important events in our lives, from births to deaths, and everything in between. Within family and cultural circles, we each have our own favourite foods and drinks that help define us as individuals.

Having diabetes or pre-diabetes does not put an end to these important functions of food. We must use our knowledge of food and nutrition in the management of diabetes and pre-diabetes to help tailor a healthy eating pattern that meets our management goals while allowing us to continue to enjoy food.

FOOD AND NUTRITION MANAGEMENT GOALS

To help put healthy eating into perspective, the American Diabetes Association (ADA) has created food and nutrition management goals that summarise all the main points to consider about healthy eating.

1) Achieve and maintain:
   — blood glucose levels in the recommended range or as close to it as is safely possible

American Diabetes Association goals that apply to specific situations:

1) For children and adolescents with type 1 diabetes, adolescents with type 2 diabetes, and pregnant and lactating women with diabetes, it is essential that you meet the nutritional needs of these unique times in your life to enable optimal growth and development.

2) For people who use insulin or medications that increase insulin production, it is important that you are educated about the safe conduct of exercise, including the prevention and treatment of hypoglycaemia, and diabetes treatment during acute illness.

   — blood pressure levels in the recommended range or as close to it as is safely possible
   — a blood cholesterol and triglyceride profile that reduces the risk of vascular diseases like heart attack, stroke, retinopathy and kidney disease.
2) Prevent or slow down the rate of development of the chronic complications of diabetes by modifying your food and nutrient intake and lifestyle.
3) Consider your individual nutrition needs, taking into account personal and cultural preferences and your willingness to make changes.

Forget about the latest fad diet or health-promoting food. Work with your dietitian to develop a healthy eating plan to maintain your pleasure of eating, and only limit food choices when indicated by the best scientific evidence.

4) Maintain your pleasure of eating by limiting food choices only when it is indicated by scientific evidence.

FAD DIETS AND FUNCTIONAL FOODS

Unfortunately, food and nutrition are plagued by fads — low fat, low carbohydrate, sugar free, gluten free and so on. Approximately 2500 'diet' books are published each year around the world, and sophisticated marketing and public relations plans are often used to sell the books and their associated products (foods, drinks and dietary supplements).

People with diabetes and pre-diabetes need to be wary of going along with the latest diet fad. The nutritional management of diabetes is complex. For most people, once you have diabetes, you need to manage it for the rest of your life. So following the latest fad is not a recipe for long-term health and wellbeing. Most fads involve the complete avoidance of a particular nutrient, food group or food. This can create a range of social issues as food and drink are often enjoyed with others, and can also lead to the development of eating disorders, which are becoming increasingly common in both women and men.

The simplest way to avoid fads is to follow the food and nutrition advice provided by reputable not-for-profit organisations like Diabetes Australia, Diabetes UK, American Diabetes Association and equivalent organisations around the world. These organisations publish reviews of scientific evidence on a regular basis (usually every 5 years). Teams of experts review published scientific evidence, rate its quality and develop comprehensive recommendations based on only the highest-quality evidence available. The technical information is then provided to health professionals so that they can provide patients with the most comprehensive and up-to-date advice. The advice is also translated into fact sheets and books like those found at local diabetes organisations.

In addition to fad diets, so-called functional foods that are low or high in the latest 'bad' or 'good' nutrient can be found in increasingly large amounts in supermarkets. Many make claims about their health benefits. While it may be tempting to try these foods, and to measure their effect on blood glucose or other indicators of diabetes management, it's important to note that the majority of the healthiest foods in the supermarket rarely make any claims at all. This is

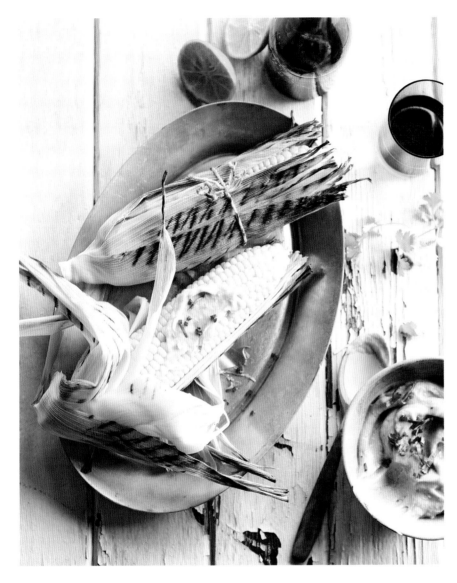

Barbecued corn
with avocado cream
is full of healthy
unsaturated fats
and dietary fibre.
Recipe page 103

partly because some of the most nutritious foods available don't come in packages or have labels. For example, most unprocessed fruits and vegetables are packed with vitamins, minerals and dietary fibre, and do not contain excessive amounts of energy (kilojoules), fat or carbohydrate. Similarly, lean meat, fish and poultry, as well as fresh grainy bread from your local baker, rarely come pre-packaged with nutrition or health claims. These core foods can be prepared in traditional ways to meet your personal and cultural needs.

We live in a multicultural society with a diverse and high-quality food supply where we enjoy a broad range of cuisines from around the world. It is possible to develop a healthy eating plan that fits within these cultural eating patterns, ensuring the enjoyment of food with a minimum disruption to family and social life. Forget about the latest fad diet or health-promoting food. Work with your dietitian to develop a healthy eating plan that is based on the latest high-quality evidence in order to maintain your pleasure of eating, and only limit food choices when indicated by the best available scientific evidence.

UNDERSTANDING THE MAJOR NUTRIENTS IN FOODS

WHILE WE EACH CHOOSE A VARIETY OF FOODS and beverages for different reasons, the biological reason that we consume foods and drinks is to obtain the nutrients our bodies need to grow, maintain good health, repair damage, do work and reproduce. The essential nutrients, or 'macronutrients', that are found in the largest amounts in foods and drinks are proteins, carbohydrates and fats. Most foods and drinks contain relatively small amounts of other essential nutrients too, including vitamins, minerals and dietary fibre.

While people talk about carbohydrate foods or protein foods, the reality is that most foods contain a mix of the macronutrients in varying proportions. For example, carbohydrate-rich foods like bread contain protein and fat, and protein-rich foods like meat contain fat. There are a few exceptions, such as refined fats, oils and sugar, but these are generally used as ingredients rather than eaten on their own.

Energy

The word energy brings to mind different concepts, from vitality, to having the 'get up and go' to do things, to the amount of kilojoules or calories in foods and drinks. Energy is all of these things.

The macronutrients protein, carbohydrate and fat are made up of four basic building blocks: carbon, hydrogen, oxygen and nitrogen. These are broken down through complex biological processes and the energy from these elements is converted to the body's universal energy currency, adenosine triphosphate (ATP). This is used to drive all the body's processes — growth, maintenance, repair and reproduction.

In the metric system, energy in foods is measured in kilojoules (kJ), which is a mandatory component in nutrition information panels on food labels. Calories (cal) are still commonly used, and can also be found in many nutrition information panels. To convert kilojoules to calories, simply divide them by 4.2.

It's worth knowing that the average estimated daily energy requirement for adult Australians and New Zealanders is 8700 kJ (2070 cal) a day. For the EU and many other parts of the world, it is 8400 kJ (2000 cal) a day. This slight difference is due to the way the requirements are estimated.

Protein

Most people know that muscles are made up of protein, and that meat is a good source of protein, but what is protein?

Proteins are chemical compounds made up of chains of amino acids, which themselves are composed of the elements carbon, hydrogen, oxygen and nitrogen. There are 20 amino acids

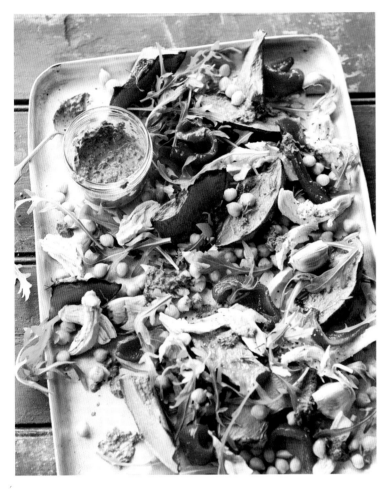

Poached chicken
with roasted pumpkin
and herb dressing
contains chicken and
chickpeas for protein.
Recipe page 165

average 80 kg adult contains about 13 kg of protein, with 43% found in muscle, 16% in blood and 15% in skin. The protein in the cells is constantly being recycled and replenished, which is one reason why we need to obtain a range of proteins from foods and drinks each day. In addition to being used to make proteins, amino acids can be used for specific purposes within our cells, such as the formation of nerve transmitters and hormones.

Amino acids can also be used as a source of energy, particularly when other sources of energy like carbohydrate and fat are restricted. In the great scheme of things, our body's top priority is to meet its energy requirements. When energy from other sources is limited, the body will break down protein to meet its needs. It does this by stripping off the nitrogen from the rest of the amino acid molecule, leaving carbon, oxygen and hydrogen skeletons to be used as fuels, just like carbohydrate, providing 17 kJ per gram of protein. When amino acids are used for energy, the nitrogen molecules are converted to urea and excreted in your urine. On the other hand, if you consume adequate carbohydrate and fat, your body spares protein from being used for energy.

that are important to humans. Nine of these amino acids (histidine, isoleucine, leucine, lysine, methionine, phenylalanine, threonine, tryptophan and valine) are considered essential because they must be obtained from foods and drinks, whereas the non-essential amino acids can be synthesised within the body. All of the proteins that are found in the body are made from these 20 amino acids.

Proteins are essential parts of the structure and function of every cell in the body. The body of an

Most people eat a variety of foods containing many different proteins. Some foods contain all nine of the essential amino acids in amounts suitable for humans and these are called complete protein foods. These include animal foods like meat, poultry, seafood, eggs and dairy foods. Soy protein is also considered to be complete. Proteins in plant foods (vegetables, grains, legumes, nuts and seeds) are rarely complete, but when they are eaten in combination with other plant foods, either at the same meal, or another time of the day, they almost always provide a complete source of protein (for example, rice and beans, or bread and peanut butter). This is one of the reasons why well-designed vegan diets can meet all of the body's nutritional requirements.

PROTEIN INTAKE

Both low and high protein intakes are detrimental to health. Low intakes can impair the immune system, will stunt the growth of children and adolescents, and will slow the healing of wounds and rates of recovery after surgery. It is possible to eat too much protein because the kidneys don't have an unlimited capacity to excrete it. The upper limit of protein consumption in humans is estimated to be 35% of energy from protein, which for a typical person consuming 8700 kJ a day would be 179 g a day. This rarely occurs under normal circumstances, but has been observed in populations where food is scarce, and people are forced to rely heavily on wild animals for food, such as rabbits, and is consequently known as rabbit starvation or *mal de caribou*. Symptoms include diarrhoea, headache, fatigue, low blood pressure and a slow heart rate, as well as a vague discomfort and hunger that can only be satisfied by consuming foods that are high in fats or carbohydrates.

The recommended dietary intake for protein is 64 g a day for men and 46 g a day for women. The most recent national nutrition survey estimated that Australian men consume 105 g of protein a day and women 78 g a day. Although men and women in the UK consume less protein than their Australian cousins (89 g and 66 g, respectively), it is still much more than the recommended dietary intake.

PROTEIN AND DIABETES

There is no evidence that people with diabetes or those at risk have different protein requirements from the general population, provided they don't have kidney disease. People with diabetes who also have chronic kidney disease are recommended to eat no more than 0.8 g of protein for each kilogram of body weight (69 g a day for an average man and 57 g a day for an average woman). There is evidence that vegetable proteins (in particular soy protein) are better for kidney function than animal proteins.

There is growing evidence that animals (including humans) have a dominant appetite for protein. If given food that is low in protein but rich in carbohydrates or fats, they will keep eating the carbohydrate- or fat-laden food until it has supplied them with enough protein. This may increase their overall energy intake, leading to weight gain. This is backed up by the world's longest weight maintenance trial, Diogenes, which found that a moderately high protein (around 22% of energy), moderate carbohydrate (around 44% of energy) and low-GI diet was the best for longer-term weight maintenance. Based on this, the optimal protein to carbohydrate ratio is about one to two. In other words, on average, aim to eat no more than 2 g of carbohydrate for every gram of protein you eat.

Glucose and insulin production

Whether a sugar or a starch, most of the carbohydrate found in foods we eat is digested in the stomach and small intestine, then absorbed into the bloodstream and, one way or another, converted to glucose.

When glucose enters the bloodstream, the pancreas releases insulin, which signals most of the body's organs and tissues to absorb the glucose from the blood. Since people with diabetes produce either no insulin (type 1) or not enough insulin (type 2), their blood glucose levels can rise too high after consuming too much of a high-carbohydrate meal or drink.

Carbohydrates

Carbohydrates are made up of carbon, hydrogen and oxygen molecules. They are largely used as an energy source by our bodies, being the preferred fuel for our brains and nervous systems, and for our exercising muscles. They have many other roles, and they add taste, texture and colour to our foods and drinks. Carbohydrates are found in plant foods and some dairy products, including milk. The three most common kinds are sugars, starches and dietary fibres.

SUGARS

The simplest form of carbohydrates are the monosaccharides (literally 'one sugar') fructose, glucose and galactose. As the name suggests, fructose is found in fruit, making up around half the carbohydrate in a typical piece, and is commonly called fruit sugar. It is also found in other foods like honey and in the sap of certain plants (for example, agave and maple trees). Glucose is also found in fruit and honey, as well as in grains and vegetables. Galactose is found in milk and other dairy products.

Two monosaccharides joined together are known as disaccharides (literally 'two sugars'). The most common varieties are sucrose, maltose and lactose. Sucrose is made up of fructose and glucose, and is the most common form of sugar in foods and drinks. It occurs naturally in fruit, but two of the best sources are sugar cane and sugar beets, which are both used to make a variety of refined sugars and are added to foods and drinks for taste, texture and colour. Maltose is made up of two units of glucose. It is found naturally in grains, such as barley, and is commonly added to foods as an ingredient. Lactose is made up of glucose and galactose, and is found in milk and yoghurt. It is also added to some foods as an ingredient.

STARCHES

Starches are made up of long chains of glucose, and are found naturally in a wide range of foods including grains, legumes, starchy vegetables, nuts and seeds. They are also added to many foods as an ingredient (for example, thickeners). There are two main kinds of starches, amylose and amylopectin. Amylose is like a string of glucose molecules that tend to line up in rows and form tight, compact clumps, whereas amylopectin is a string of glucose molecules with lots of branching points — a bit like a tree.

Eating more fruits, vegetables, legumes and whole grains is the best way to meet your daily fibre requirements. Dietary guidelines recommend we eat the following amounts each day.

FRUITS:
2 plus serves a day
A serve is one medium or two small pieces, or 1 cup of tinned fruit.

VEGETABLES:
5 to 6 serves a day
A serve is 1 cup of salad vegetables, or ½ cup of other vegetables or legumes.

WHOLE GRAINS:
3 to 6 serves a day
A serve is ½–⅔ cup of breakfast cereal, 1 slice of grainy bread, ½ grainy roll, ½ cup of cooked brown rice, wholemeal (whole-wheat) pasta, noodles, barley, buckwheat, semolina, burghul (bulgur) or quinoa.

You can also add extra fibre to meals and recipes by sprinkling on bran flakes, psyllium husks, dried fruit, nuts or seeds.

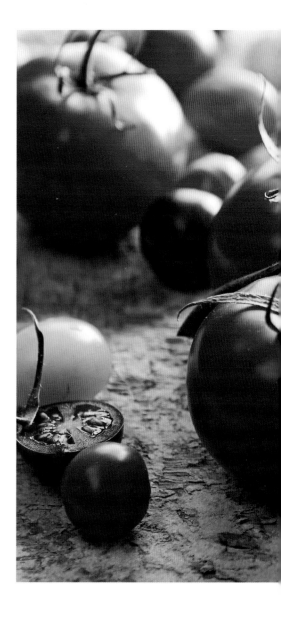

DIETARY FIBRES

Most dietary fibres are a form of carbohydrate, but they do not raise blood glucose levels. Dietary fibres come mainly from plants and they are the poorly digested portions that pass through into the large intestine and provide much of the bulk in our stools.

There are a number of ways of classifying the different types of fibre. One of the most popular systems is based on whether or not the fibre is soluble in water.

- Water-soluble fibres include gums (for example, agar), fructans (for example, inulin), mucilages (for example, psyllium) and pectins. They are found in a wide range of foods including fruits, vegetables, legumes and some grains.
- Water-insoluble fibres include cellulose, hemicellulose and lignins. They are mostly found in vegetables, wheat and other whole grains, nuts and seeds.

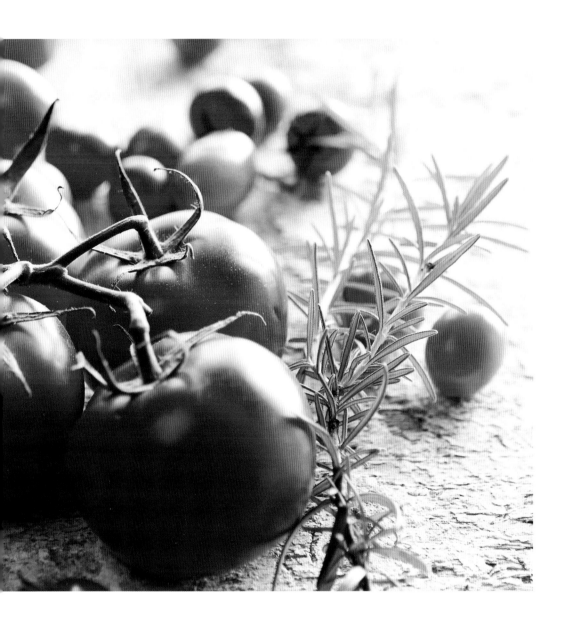

The different types of dietary fibres have different effects on our health.

- Soluble dietary fibre may help to reduce blood cholesterol levels and modulate blood glucose levels (whether it does so or not depends in part on the degree of food processing and how much you eat).
- Insoluble dietary fibre primarily helps with laxation, which in turn may decrease the risk of constipation, haemorrhoids and colo-rectal (bowel) cancer.

The recommended intake of total fibre each day is 25 g for women and 30 g for men. At this point in time, there aren't any specific recommendations for the different types of fibre.

Australia's most recent national nutrition survey found that, on average, women eat 21 g of fibre a day and men eat 25 g a day. So on average, Australians eat 4 to 5 g less fibre each day than recommended. In the UK, women consume 12.8 g a day and men consume 14.8 g a day, falling well short of the target.

LOW-GI FOODS

Dense wholegrain bread

Authentic sourdough bread

Barley

Quinoa

Pasta and noodles

Pearl couscous

Doongara rice

Legumes

Bran

Rolled (porridge) oats

Natural muesli

Most fruits and vegetables
  (except melons and
  most potatoes)

Milk

Yoghurt

MEDIUM-GI FOODS

Raisins

Rice (basmati, arborio and
  long-grain)

Carisma potatoes

Soft drinks

Sweet biscuits and cakes

HIGH-GI FOODS

White bread

Potatoes

Jasmine rice

Many breakfast cereals (e.g.
  flaked corn and puffed rice)

Sport drinks

Confectionery

Rice malt syrup

Most crackers

Most savoury snacks

Chips (fries)

GLYCAEMIC INDEX (GI)

Essentially all sugars and starches in food are digested, absorbed and metabolised into glucose. However, some foods break down quickly during digestion, are absorbed quickly and don't require further metabolism, so they cause the glucose in the blood to increase rapidly. On the other hand, some foods break down slowly during digestion or take longer to be absorbed or metabolised, and so the glucose is released gradually into the bloodstream.

The glycaemic index (GI), is a number between one and 100 that provides a way of estimating how fast the body is going to digest, absorb and metabolise carbohydrate-containing foods, and how high blood glucose levels will rise as a consequence. Simply, foods that are digested, absorbed and metabolised into glucose quickly have a high GI, and those that are digested, absorbed and metabolised into glucose slowly have a low GI. By definition, high-GI foods and drinks have a GI value of 70 and above, medium-GI foods and drinks have a GI value between 56 and 69, and low-GI foods and drinks have a GI value of 55 and under.

The GI of a food is measured in a group of 10 or more healthy people following an internationally standardised procedure. Each person is usually given a 50 g portion of available carbohydrate (sugars and starches, but not dietary fibre). Their blood glucose levels are then measured every 15 minutes for the next 2 hours. This process is followed for both a standard food (glucose or white bread) and a test food, on two separate days. The blood glucose levels from both days are plotted on a graph, the dots are joined to create a blood glucose curve, and the area under the blood glucose curve is calculated using computer software. The result for the test food is divided by the result for pure glucose to derive the GI value, which is simply a percentage.

GLYCAEMIC LOAD (GL)

Because we do not necessarily consume 50 g of carbohydrate every time we have a carbohydrate-containing food or drink, the concept of glycaemic load (GL) was developed. To calculate GL, multiply the GI by the amount of carbohydrate found in a typical serving of food and divide the result by 100. For example, a typical slice of white bread has a GI of 71 and contains 15 g of carbohydrate. Therefore, its glycaemic load is $71 \times 15 \div 100 = 10.6$. If you, like many people, eat two slices of bread as part of a sandwich, the overall GL of this meal is 21.

For optimal health, the average adult should aim to consume less than 100 units of GL in a typical day. A meal has a low GL if the value is less than 30, and it has a high GL if the value is greater than 60. There is very good evidence from clinical trials that the GL of a food or meal is the best predictor of a person's blood glucose and insulin levels — better than the GI or amount of available carbohydrate alone.

DIABETES, GI AND GL

While the glycaemic index and glycaemic load may sound like complicated concepts, using them is relatively easy. Simply swap healthy low-GI foods and drinks for regular high-GI varieties within the same food group or category, using the 'Swap it, don't stop it' approach. For example, a typical slice of white or wholemeal (whole-wheat) bread has a high GI. Rather than stop eating bread altogether, simply swap it for a healthier low-GI alternative like authentic sourdough, dense multigrain or wholegrain varieties.

If you select the lowest-GI food within a food group or category, you are also most likely choosing the one that has the lowest GL, because foods are usually grouped together due to their similar macronutrient content (e.g. their carbohydrate or protein content).

Using this approach, there's very powerful evidence from clinical trials in people with diabetes that you can decrease your HbA1c by an average of 0.5 percentage points above and beyond what you would achieve by following a healthy diet alone. In addition, it may also decrease your risk of having a hypo (if you use insulin or other insulin-raising medications), which is important from a quality of life perspective.

Fibre and GI

It's worth noting that just because a food is high in fibre, it does not necessarily have a low GI. There are two main reasons why this is the case:

1) Soluble fibre may lower the GI of some foods, but they need to contain appreciable amounts, and the size of the fibre molecules needs to be large enough to have an effect. Excessive processing decreases the size of fibre molecules.

2) Insoluble fibre can help slow the rate of carbohydrate digestion or absorption if the fibre is largely intact. Adding highly processed fibres usually does not have the same effect.

HOW MUCH CARBOHYDRATE SHOULD I EAT?

Now that you know about the different kinds of carbohydrates and how to gauge their effect on your blood glucose levels, you are probably wondering how much you are able to eat. The answer depends on a whole range of factors, including your body size, age, gender, level of physical activity, personal food preferences, cultural background and the amount and type of insulin or diabetes medication that you are taking.

It's worth remembering that before insulin was identified, isolated and made commercially available, most people with diabetes used to have to eat very low carbohydrate diets in order to stay alive. While these diets did prolong life, they were extremely unpleasant. After insulin became commonly available, people with diabetes began to include carbohydrate foods in their diets again, but they still generally restricted how much they ate.

By the 1970s, ongoing research indicated that cardiovascular disease was a leading cause of death in the general population as well as in people with diabetes. Because fat has the most powerful effect on blood cholesterol levels, which are in turn a major risk factor for cardiovascular disease, people were advised to consume lower-fat (in particular lower saturated fat), higher-carbohydrate diets.

Over the past few decades, diabetes organisations around the world have recommended that people with diabetes consume 45 to 60% of their energy (kilojoules) from carbohydrates, which is consistent with healthy eating guidelines for the general public. For a typical healthy adult consuming 8700 kJ each day, who is not overweight and participates in light physical activity, this would equate to between 230 g and 470 g of carbohydrate each day. The most recent Australian Health Survey indicates that the average adult consumes 222 g of carbohydrate a day, or 43.5% of energy, which is close to the bottom end of the general recommendation. In other words, most Australians don't consume a high-carbohydrate diet. In the UK, the most recent National Diet and Nutrition Survey indicates that the average adult consumes roughly the same amount of carbohydrate (221.5 g) as their Australian cousins, but it is a higher percentage of their energy intake (47% of kilojoules), which puts them close to the bottom end of the recommended range.

Ongoing research has shown that a variety of eating patterns, including lower-carbohydrate, higher-protein and Mediterranean-style diets, can all be effective in decreasing HbA1c in people with diabetes by between 0.12 and 0.47 percentage points, depending on the eating pattern, if they are followed for 6 to 18 months. We don't really know what happens after that. Most long-term studies (that is, more than 2 years) show that people slowly but surely go back to eating what they used to eat. It makes sense — you have acquired your food preferences over the course of a lifetime, and following a completely different eating plan from what you are used to is a difficult task no matter how strong your willpower.

Diabetes organisations have recommended that people with diabetes consume 45 to 60% of their energy from carbohydrates, which is consistent with healthy eating guidelines for the general public.

Rather than trying to follow any particular regimen, you are arguably better off eating and drinking less of the foods and drinks you currently enjoy, and swapping to healthier alternatives. That way you can continue to enjoy food with your family and friends for the rest of your days. This is where having your own registered or accredited dietitian is important. They can help design a personalised eating plan that meets all of your nutrition needs at an affordable price, and that you can live with in the long term.

CARB COUNTING

Whatever carbohydrate you choose to eat, it is important for most people with diabetes to match their insulin or blood glucose lowering medication with the amount of carbohydrate they eat and the time that they eat it. In general, three main meals a day that contain carbohydrate foods are adequate for most adults. Children, adolescents, athletes of any age, and adults on certain insulin regimens or diabetes medications may need carbohydrate-containing snacks in between meals. Discuss this with your dietitian or doctor if you are not sure.

There are a number of commonly used systems for estimating the amount of carbohydrate in foods so that insulin and medication requirements can be matched. While there are pros and cons for each method, research has shown that the actual method used doesn't really matter. The most important factor is what works best for you in the long term.

When first diagnosed, most people with type 1 diabetes are taught how to count the grams of carbohydrate, or to use 10 g carbohydrate portions or 15 g carbohydrate exchange systems, to estimate the amount of carbohydrate in their foods and drinks. Adults with type 1 diabetes who use carb-counting techniques can lower their HbA1c by 0.4 percentage points and there is some evidence that they may decrease their risk of having a hypo.

When first diagnosed, people with type 2 diabetes are also usually provided with lots of information and advice to help them evenly spread out the amount of carbohydrate they eat throughout the day. They are not usually taught how to count carbs, or how to use carbohydrate portions or carbohydrate exchanges, unless they are going to commence using intensive insulin regimens.

Fat facts

Foods that are high in fat generally contain the most kilojoules. This is because each gram of fat provides 37 kJ, whereas protein and carbohydrate (including sugars) provide less than half that amount of energy (17 kJ per gram of protein and 16.5 kJ per gram of carbohydrate). One easy way to reduce your total energy intake is to look for lower-fat versions of the foods that you already eat. However, make sure that the fat hasn't been replaced by highly refined carbohydrate (starches or sugars) as they may help reduce the kilojoule content, but have unwanted effects on blood glucose and insulin levels.

Fats

Fats are an essential nutrient and they are also an enjoyable part of healthy eating. They:
• form the structure of all the body's cells
• are used in the manufacture of bile and sex hormones
• insulate our body against cold and protect our organs
• are the main source of the fat-soluble vitamins (vitamins A, D, E and K)
• are a concentrated source of energy (37 kJ per gram) in foods
• are a major source of stored energy within the body
• carry many of the pleasant flavours associated with foods.

Most of the fats we consume, whether they are from animal or vegetable sources, are in the form of triglycerides when we eat them. Triglycerides are fat molecules that are composed of three fatty acids joined to a glycerol (a sugar alcohol) backbone. Fatty acids themselves are chains of hydrogen and carbon, with an acid group at one end. The digestive organs break down fats into free fatty acids and they are absorbed into the intestinal cells, reassembled and then eventually released into the bloodstream.

Because fat has so many important uses, a fat-free diet is both undesirable and unnecessary. It is possible to significantly change the total fat content of your diet from low to high fat (depending on your personal preferences and particular needs) without detrimentally affecting your health — provided that you eat the right kind of fat.

There are four main kinds of fat in our diets: saturated fat, trans fat, mono-unsaturated fat and polyunsaturated fat. Collectively, mono-unsaturated and polyunsaturated fats are called unsaturated fats. The major sources of the various kinds of fats are listed opposite.

Of course, foods and ingredients are not pure sources of any particular kind of fat — they contain a mixture of different kinds of fatty acids. It is much more practical to swap from high saturated fat and trans fat foods and ingredients to lower equivalents, rather than trying to strictly avoid any particular one of them.

Major sources of dietary fat

SATURATED FATS

Spreads
- *Butter*
- *Solid cooking margarines*

Oils/fat
- *Coconut oil*
- *Copha (white vegetable shortening)*
- *Ghee*
- *Lard*
- *Palm oil*
- *Palm kernel oil*
- *Solid frying oils*

Dairy fat
- *Cheese*
- *Cream*
- *Full-cream ice cream, yoghurt and milk*
- *Sour cream*

Meat fat
- *Fat around and in meat*
- *Skin on poultry*

Miscellaneous
- *Commercial biscuits*
- *Most cakes, pastries and chips (fries)*
- *Many takeaway foods*

TRANS FATS

Spreads
- *Butter*
- *Cheap unbranded margarines*
- *Cooking margarines*

Oils/fat
- *Some cooking fats used for deep-frying and in some baked goods*
- *Copha (white vegetable shortening)*

Dairy fat
- *Cheese*

Meat fat
- *Fat around and in meat*
- *Fried chicken*

Miscellaneous
- *Some commercial biscuits, cakes, pastries and chips (fries)*
- *Takeaway foods*

MONO-UNSATURATED FATS

Spreads
- *Canola, olive oil or sunola-based margarines*

Oils
- *Olive*
- *Canola*
- *Peanut*
- *Avocado*
- *Macadamia*

Fruit
- *Avocado*

Nuts and nut spreads
- *Peanuts*
- *Cashews*
- *Almonds*
- *Hazelnuts*
- *Macadamias*
- *Pecans*
- *Pistachios*

Seeds
- *Sesame seeds*
- *Sunflower seeds*
- *Pepitas (pumpkin seeds)*

POLYUNSATURATED FATS

Spreads
- *Polyunsaturated margarines*

Oils
- *Safflower*
- *Sunflower*
- *Canola*
- *Soya bean*
- *Corn*
- *Sesame*
- *Cottonseed*
- *Linseed (flaxseed)*
- *Grapeseed*
- *Fish oils*

Fish
- *Herring*
- *Salmon*
- *Tuna*
- *Mackerel*
- *Sardines*
- *Swordfish*
- *Shellfish*

Nuts and nut spreads
- *Walnuts*
- *Brazil nuts*
- *Pine nuts*

Seeds
- *Linseeds (flaxseeds)*
- *Chia seeds*
- *Sesame seeds*
- *Sunflower seeds*
- *Pepitas (pumpkin seeds)*

Unsaturated fats can help lower LDL cholesterol and raise HDL cholesterol, decreasing your risk of cardiovascular disease. It is therefore important that you eat some of these good fats every day.

SATURATED FAT AND TRANS FAT

Frequent consumption of large amounts of foods and ingredients high in saturated fat is not good for you because they are the kind that raise the 'bad' LDL cholesterol, which can block blood vessels, thereby increasing your risk of cardiovascular disease.

Like saturated fat, trans fat increases the amount of LDL cholesterol in the blood, but it also lowers the 'good' HDL cholesterol. So the overall effect is even worse for your health than saturated fat.

To reduce the amount of saturated fat and to limit the amount of trans fat you eat:
• choose lean meat and trim off fat before cooking
• remove the skin from chicken (where possible, before cooking)
• limit your use of butter, cheap unbranded margarine, hard cooking margarine, lard, dripping, cream and sour cream
• choose reduced- or low-fat milk, yoghurt, ice cream and custard
• limit the quantity of cheese you eat, and choose reduced-fat varieties
• limit pastries, cakes, puddings, chocolate and cream biscuits to special occasions
• limit pre-packaged biscuits, savoury packet snacks, cakes, frozen and convenience meals
• limit the consumption of processed deli meats and sausages
• avoid fried takeaway foods such as chips (fries), fried chicken and battered fish; choose skinless barbecued chicken and grilled (broiled) fish instead
• avoid pies, sausage rolls and pasties
• choose tomato- and soy-based sauces rather than creamy sauces, and avoid creamy-style soups.

MONO-UNSATURATED FAT AND POLYUNSATURATED FAT

Unsaturated fats can help lower LDL cholesterol levels and raise HDL cholesterol, decreasing your risk of cardiovascular disease. It is therefore important that you eat some of these good fats every day.

To increase the amount of mono-unsaturated and polyunsaturated fat you eat:
• stir-fry meat and vegetables with garlic or chilli in peanut, sesame, soya bean or canola oil or oil spray
• dress a salad or steamed vegetables with a little olive oil and lemon juice or vinegar

- sprinkle sesame seeds on steamed vegetables
- eat bread that has linseeds (flaxseeds) added and spread it with a little olive oil or canola margarine
- snack on a handful of unsalted nuts, or add some to a stir-fry or salad
- spread avocado on toast and sandwiches, or add it to a salad
- eat more fish (at least three times a week).

Plant sterols and stanols

Plant sterols and stanols are naturally occurring ingredients that can help reduce the absorption of cholesterol from food. They are found in small amounts in:

- nuts, seeds and legumes
- vegetable oils
- breads and cereals
- fruits and vegetables.

They are also available in more concentrated amounts in some margarines. When eaten in the specified amounts (typically 25 g per day, equivalent to 1 tablespoon of margarine), plant sterols and stanols may lower blood cholesterol levels by as much as 10 to 15%.

CHOLESTEROL IN FOODS

Cholesterol is a special kind of fat that is only found in foods that come from animals, such as meat and dairy products. The main nutrients in food that cause LDL cholesterol levels to rise are saturated and trans fats, not cholesterol. However, if you eat a diet high in saturated fat, eating high-cholesterol foods can raise some people's blood cholesterol levels by an additional 10 to 20%.

If your blood cholesterol levels are high despite reducing your consumption of foods and ingredients that are high in saturated and trans fats, increasing your consumption of unsaturated fats, and using plant sterols and stanols, you may wish to reduce your cholesterol intake to less than 200 mg a day.

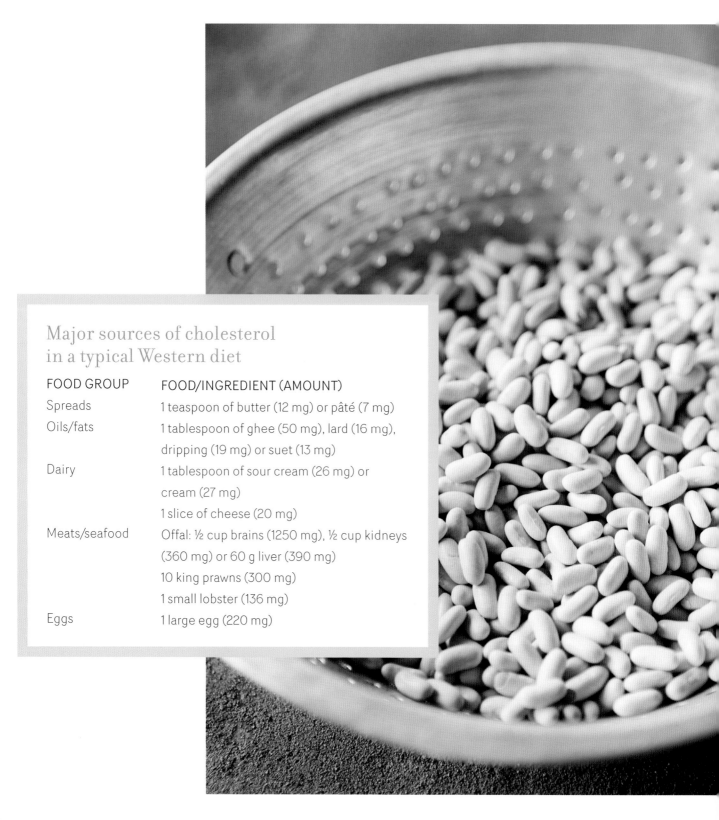

Major sources of cholesterol in a typical Western diet

FOOD GROUP	FOOD/INGREDIENT (AMOUNT)
Spreads	1 teaspoon of butter (12 mg) or pâté (7 mg)
Oils/fats	1 tablespoon of ghee (50 mg), lard (16 mg), dripping (19 mg) or suet (13 mg)
Dairy	1 tablespoon of sour cream (26 mg) or cream (27 mg)
	1 slice of cheese (20 mg)
Meats/seafood	Offal: ½ cup brains (1250 mg), ½ cup kidneys (360 mg) or 60 g liver (390 mg)
	10 king prawns (300 mg)
	1 small lobster (136 mg)
Eggs	1 large egg (220 mg)

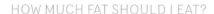

HOW MUCH FAT SHOULD I EAT?

Because the different kinds of fat are found in such a broad range of foods, it is essential that we eat a variety of foods in the right balance. A good guide is to avoid trans fats as much as possible, and for every gram of saturated fat you eat, eat 2 g of unsaturated fat. This means that you do not have to avoid all foods and ingredients that are high in saturated fat — it's all about balance.

The amount of fat you should eat depends on a number of factors like your age (low-fat diets are not recommended for infants and young children), your weight (lower-fat diets are sometimes recommended if you are trying to lose weight), your level of physical activity, and your cultural background (some cultures like the Japanese traditionally have a low-fat diet, whereas people from the Mediterranean traditionally eat a higher-fat diet). For personalised advice, see your dietitian.

Carbohydrates and cholesterol

While fats are the primary nutrient of interest when it comes to examining blood cholesterol levels, carbohydrate-containing foods also have a role. For example, legumes, fruits, vegetables and oats contain certain kinds of fibre that may help lower blood cholesterol levels by binding it in the gut. As well as dietary fibre, there is growing evidence that the kind of carbohydrate that we eat also has an effect on our blood cholesterol levels.

A recent analysis of 28 randomised controlled trials provided high-level evidence that high-fibre, low-GI diets can significantly reduce total and LDL cholesterol levels, independent of weight loss. Healthy low-GI diets are thought to lower blood cholesterol levels by decreasing insulin secretion, thereby reducing the activity of the key enzyme involved in cholesterol synthesis.

Simple ways to reduce your salt intake

- When shopping, look for products that are 'salt reduced' or have 'no added salt'.
- Reduce or omit salt in cooking.
- Avoid sea salt, rock salt, garlic salt, chicken salt, etc. as they are not suitable substitutes for salt.
- Instead of using salt for flavour, use spices such as pepper, chilli, curry, mustard, paprika and cardamom.
- Add flavour with herbs like parsley, basil, oregano, chives, rosemary, coriander (cilantro), mint, sage, thyme, tarragon and marjoram.
- Add lemon juice, onions, garlic, ginger, spring onions (scallions), vinegar, wine or salt-reduced stock for extra flavour.
- Don't put salt on the table to add to food.

Salt or sodium

With all the negative information in the media about salt or sodium, it's easy to forget that it is an essential nutrient. Sodium has a number of important functions in the body, including maintaining fluid balance within the cells and organs, and helping to regulate acidity, and it is an essential component of nerve impulse transmission.

Dietary guidelines around the world recommend that people eat less, or limit, added salt and salty foods. The salt they are referring to is sodium chloride, the most common salt added to foods. It has been used as a condiment by humans for many thousands of years. As well as enhancing flavour, salt has other important roles including acting as a preservative and affecting a food's texture. Salt is approximately 40% sodium and 60% chloride.

The main reason why we need to eat less salt is that consumption of large amounts raises blood pressure in many people and in turn may increase the risk of cardiovascular disease. High salt intakes are also associated with an increased risk of developing stomach cancer. The World Health Organisation (WHO) currently recommends that adults consume less than 2 g (2000 mg) of sodium each day, which is equivalent to less than 5.1 g (1 teaspoon) of added salt.

Surveys from around the world indicate that most people eat more salt than is required for good health. The most recent Australian Health Survey indicates that the average Australian adult consumes over 2.4 g (2430 mg) of sodium each day, equivalent to over 6.2 g of salt. The most recent UK survey indicates that the average British adult consumes

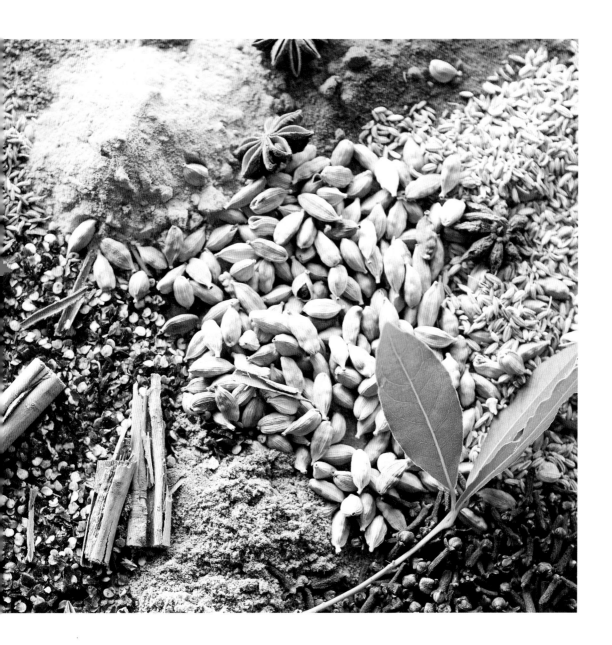

over 3.2 g (3240 mg) of sodium each day, equivalent to over 8.1 grams of salt. In the Australian survey, sodium was defined as that which occurs naturally in food or was added during food processing and does not include what is added during food preparation at home or at the table, so for most Australians the result is likely to be an underestimation. The UK results are based on the excretion of sodium in the urine, and are therefore likely to be more accurate.

While advice to reduce the amount of sodium in the diet makes good sense for most people, it is important to remember that we do not need to avoid all sodium. Too little sodium may not be good for our health either. A recent large study of adults living in 17 countries found that both lower (less than 3 g) and higher (more than 6 g) sodium intake was associated with an increased risk of major cardiovascular events like heart attack and stroke, and that an intake in the middle was associated with the least risk.

There is also evidence in people with diabetes that very low salt intakes may increase the risk of cardiovascular disease. Too little of a particular nutrient really can be just as detrimental to your health as too much.

While consuming too much sodium will raise some people's blood pressure, relatively higher intakes of potassium are associated with lower blood pressure and a lower risk of cardiovascular disease.

Potassium

Potassium is another essential nutrient with a number of important functions within the body. These include maintaining fluid balance within the cells and organs, and helping to regulate acidity. Potassium is also part of the hydrochloric acid found in the stomach that is necessary for the proper digestion of foods.

One of the reasons dietary guidelines around the world advise us to eat more vegetables and fruits is because they are all good sources of potassium.

The best sources of potassium include:
- leafy green vegetables, such as bok choy (pak choy), silverbeet (Swiss chard) and English spinach
- vine fruits, such as tomatoes, cucumbers, zucchini (courgette), eggplant (aubergine) and pumpkin (winter squash)
- root vegetables, such as potatoes, sweet potatoes and carrots.

Moderately good sources of potassium include:
- beans (for example, baked beans and kidney beans)
- peas
- dried fruits
- fresh fruits, such as apples, oranges and bananas.

Milk, yoghurt and unprocessed meats also contain potassium, although not as much as vegetables and fruits.

While consuming too much sodium will raise some people's blood pressure, relatively higher intakes of potassium are associated with lower blood pressure and a lower risk of cardiovascular disease. What this really means is that the ratio of sodium to potassium is what really counts when it comes to blood pressure and cardiovascular disease risk. The WHO recommends we should aim to consume no more sodium than potassium. In terms of absolute intakes of potassium, men should aim to consume 3800 mg and women 2800 mg each day.

Calcium

Calcium is the most abundant mineral in the body, as it is one of the essential components in bones and teeth. In addition to this essential role, calcium is also involved in the contraction of the muscles (including the heart), nerve impulse transmission, blood clotting and immune function. Needless to say, we cannot live without it.

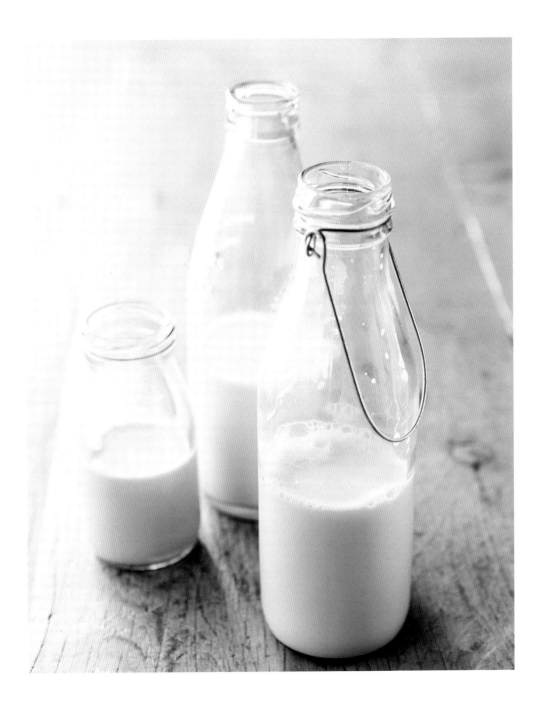

Calcium also has an effect on blood pressure, as both sodium and calcium excretion are linked in the kidneys. The more calcium you consume, the more sodium you excrete in your urine, and vice versa. This is one likely reason why consumption of dairy foods is linked to decreased risk of cardiovascular disease. While calcium is found predominantly in mammalian milk, fortified soy beverages and dairy foods, moderate amounts can also be obtained from fish that have edible bones (for example, sardines and salmon), legumes and certain nuts (for example, almonds and walnuts). Eating two to three serves of reduced- or low-fat dairy products or alternatives each day is currently recommended.

Younger men and women should aim to consume 1000 mg of calcium each day. Older men and women should consume 1300 mg each day to reduce the risk of developing osteoporosis.

CHOOSING THE RIGHT DRINKS

FOR OPTIMAL HEALTH AND WELLBEING, WE NEED between 35 and 45 ml of fluid for every kilogram of body weight each day, depending on our gender, level of physical activity, body composition and the weather. As an example, the average Australian woman weighs 71 kg and the average man 86 kg, so a typical woman needs 2.5 to 3.2 litres, and a man needs 3.0 to 3.9 litres of fluid each day. All fluids do not need to come from drinks, however, as around 750 ml comes from our food and a further 250 ml comes from the metabolism of food. So, on average, women should aim to drink 1.5 to 2.2 litres and men should aim to drink 2.0 to 2.9 litres each day.

With so many drinks to choose from, it can be confusing to know which option is best. Like most things, it depends on your personal circumstances and the occasion.

Water
It goes without saying that plain water is the best drink to quench your thirst: it is the most refreshing and provides zero kilojoules, plus a few minerals. Pure water doesn't have any taste, although the minerals that are sometimes found in water naturally, or that are added (for example, fluoride), can affect its flavour. If water flavour is an issue for you, try using a water purifier or adding a slice or two of lemon or lime.

Depending on the source, mineral water usually contains small amounts of sodium, potassium, calcium and magnesium, and is a suitable alternative to plain water for people with diabetes and those at risk.

Diet soft drinks
People with diabetes and those at risk can enjoy diet or low-joule soft drinks occasionally, but arguably they should not consume them on a daily basis. This is because carbonated beverages are acidic and frequent consumption may increase the risk of developing tooth decay. However, these types of soft drinks have no effect on blood glucose levels and they provide very few kilojoules. There is some good evidence that substituting regular soft drinks with diet or low-joule varieties will help some people to lose weight.

It is important to note, though, that diet soft drinks have also been associated with an increased risk of type 2 diabetes in observational studies. The association is likely due to what we call confounding, which means that people who regularly consume these types of drinks also have other health habits that are likely to increase their risk. However, higher-quality research is required before we can know this for certain.

Fruit juices and fruit drinks

Fruit juices and fruit drinks can also be enjoyed occasionally, but ideally not on a daily basis. They are a source of kilojoules, vitamin C, dietary fibre and carbohydrate. On average, they provide 400 kJ per 250 ml serve and are an important source of vitamin C, providing on average 113 mg in a 250 ml serve, which is more than twice the RDI of 45 mg per day. Most fruit juice contains a small amount of dietary fibre, but higher-fibre varieties are becoming increasingly common.

Fruit juices and drinks are acidic and are also a source of fermentable carbohydrate for cariogenic bacteria, so frequent consumption of these drinks may increase the risk of developing tooth decay.

Fruit juices and drinks raise blood glucose levels in people with diabetes. On average, they provide 22 g of carbohydrate per 250 ml serve. Fruit juices made from low-GI fruit and most fruit drinks have a low glycaemic index (GI), while a 250 ml serve of most varieties has a medium glycaemic load (GL).

Perhaps surprisingly, fruit juices and drinks are suitable for treating a person who is having a hypo, despite the fact that most varieties have a low GI.

Fruit juices and fruit drinks are associated with an increased risk of type 2 diabetes in observational studies. This association may be due to their kilojoule content, which may contribute to weight gain, and glycaemic load, which may contribute to pancreatic stress. Higher-quality research is also required to prove this association.

Regular sugar-sweetened soft drinks

Ideally, people who have diabetes and those who are at risk should save sugar-sweetened beverages for special occasions. Like fruit juices and fruit drinks, sugar-sweetened soft drinks are acidic and their consumption is associated with an increased risk of tooth decay.

On average, a 250 ml glass of sugar-sweetened soft drink provides 440 kJ and 27 g of carbohydrate (2 exchanges). Most soft drinks have a medium GI and a medium to high glycaemic load. Consequently, they will cause blood glucose levels to rise in people with diabetes.

Like fruit juices and fruit drinks, regular soft drinks are suitable for treating hypoglycaemia, even though most varieties have a medium GI.

> ## One standard drink equals
> - 100 ml wine
> - 285 ml regular or low-carb beer
> - 425 ml low-alcohol beer
> - 250 ml cider
> - 30 ml spirits
> - 60 ml fortified wine

Sugar-sweetened soft drinks have been associated with an increased risk of type 2 diabetes in observational studies. Like fruit juices and drinks, this association may be due to the kilojoule content of these drinks, which may contribute to weight gain, and their glycaemic load, which may contribute to pancreatic stress.

Alcohol

While alcohol is not an essential nutrient, it is nevertheless enjoyed by the majority of adults living in Australia and the UK. Alcohol provides 29 kJ of energy for every gram consumed — second only to fats in energy density. When consumed, alcohol is very rapidly absorbed into the bloodstream from the stomach and small intestine, as it doesn't require any digestion, and can consequently bring on the familiar feelings of euphoria within minutes if it is consumed on an empty stomach.

Alcohol is metabolised in the liver, but there is a limit to how much it can handle — about 15 grams (or 1½ standard drinks) an hour — so excess amounts can rapidly build up in the blood if you drink more than one or two standard drinks an hour. Also, while the liver prefers to use fatty acids for fuel, it is forced to use alcohol as a fuel when it is around. This means there can be a build-up of fatty acids in the liver and an increase in triglycerides in the blood when alcohol is consumed in excessive amounts.

On the positive side, some alcoholic beverages like red wine contain an antioxidant that may slow the development of atherosclerosis (the hardening of the arteries), decreasing the risk of cardiovascular disease. There is also some evidence that a moderate amount of alcohol (one to two standard drinks per day) may protect people from developing type 2 diabetes.

In people who already have diabetes, a moderate amount of alcohol consumed with food has very little effect on blood glucose levels — in fact some studies have shown it can reduce blood glucose levels if it is consumed just before or with a meal, which may be beneficial under certain circumstances. The effect of different types of alcoholic drinks on blood glucose levels is discussed in the table opposite.

ALCOHOL AND DIABETES

Most people with diabetes can safely enjoy alcohol in moderation, which is generally considered to be no more than two standard drinks on any day, whether you are a man or a woman.

Alcohol, carbohydrate and kilojoule content of popular drinks

BEER

285 ML GLASS OF BEER	ALCOHOL (G)	CARBOHYDRATE (G)	KILOJOULES
Regular beer	11.1	5.7	433
Low-carb beer	9.7	2.6	345
Low-alcohol beer	2	3.2	121

Low-alcohol beers are the best choice if you want to limit your total alcohol, carbohydrate and kilojoule intake. Most people will not notice any difference in blood glucose levels between the different types of beer, provided they are consumed in moderation, because all beers contain a relatively small amount of carbohydrate.

WINE

100 ML GLASS OF WINE	ALCOHOL (G)	CARBOHYDRATE (G)	KILOJOULES
White wine	9	1.1	276
Red wine	9.5	0	282
Dessert wine	8.5	10	410
Reduced-alcohol wine (white)	5.2	1.1	170
Reduced-alcohol wine (red)	5.2	0	153

Reduced-alcohol wines are the best choice overall when it comes to alcohol, carbohydrate and kilojoules. Like beer, most wine has such a small amount of carbohydrate that it will have a negligible effect on blood glucose levels if consumed in moderation. The exception is dessert wine, which is higher in total carbohydrate and kilojoules.

CIDER

250 ML GLASS OF CIDER	ALCOHOL (G)	CARBOHYDRATE (G)	KILOJOULES
Apple (dry)	9.3	7.8	403
Apple (sweet)	9.3	17.3	553
Pear	10.0	13.8	488

Cider is higher in carbohydrate and kilojoules than most other alcoholic beverages, with the exception of dessert wines.

SPIRITS

1 SHOT (30 ML) OF SPIRITS	ALCOHOL (G)	CARBOHYDRATE (G)	KILOJOULES
Gin	8.8	0	256
Rum	8.8	0	255
Vodka	8.8	0	255
Whisky	8.8	0	254

Spirits, if consumed straight or neat, provide no carbohydrate and all have essentially the same amount of kilojoules. Many people choose to consume them with mixers, however. Soda water, mineral waters and diet soft drinks provide essentially no added carbohydrate or kilojoules and are an appropriate choice for many people watching their weight.

Healthy nibbles

Of course, the nibbles that usually accompany the drinks at most special occasions need to be considered as well, as they may affect blood glucose levels and ultimately your weight. Delicious and nutritious examples include:

SAVOURY SNACKS

Ryvita

Vita-Weat

Pitta and other flatbreads
(cut into strips or
wedges)

Authentic sourdough
(cut into strips or bite-
sized squares)

Nuts and seeds

VEGETABLES AND FRUITS

Fresh raw vegetable sticks

Salads

Pickled vegetables

Baked vegetables

Fruit platters

Fresh fruit salad

Dried fruit (e.g. dates, figs,
apricots)

DIPS AND SAUCES

Hummus

Salsa-based dips

Flavoured cottage cheese

Soy-based sauces (e.g. oyster
sauce, teriyaki sauce)

Chilli, tomato or barbecue sauce

There is no simple way to determine what kind of alcoholic beverage is best for you. Along with the taste, the amount of alcohol, carbohydrate and kilojoules contained in alcoholic beverages are all important factors to consider when choosing a drink.

The number of standard drinks must be listed on all alcoholic beverages sold in Australia and New Zealand (not the UK). Unfortunately, the kilojoules and carbohydrates are not currently required, but they are starting to appear on some brands of beer.

SPECIAL CONDITIONS FOR PEOPLE WITH DIABETES

You should take extra care when drinking alcohol if you are taking sulphonylureas (for example, Amaryl, Minidiab, Diamicron and Daonil), meglitinides (for example, Prandin and Starlix), or insulin, as the alcohol and the medication can interact and cause a hypo. If you are not sure, ask your doctor, diabetes educator or pharmacist about the effects that alcohol is likely to have on your particular diabetes medication.

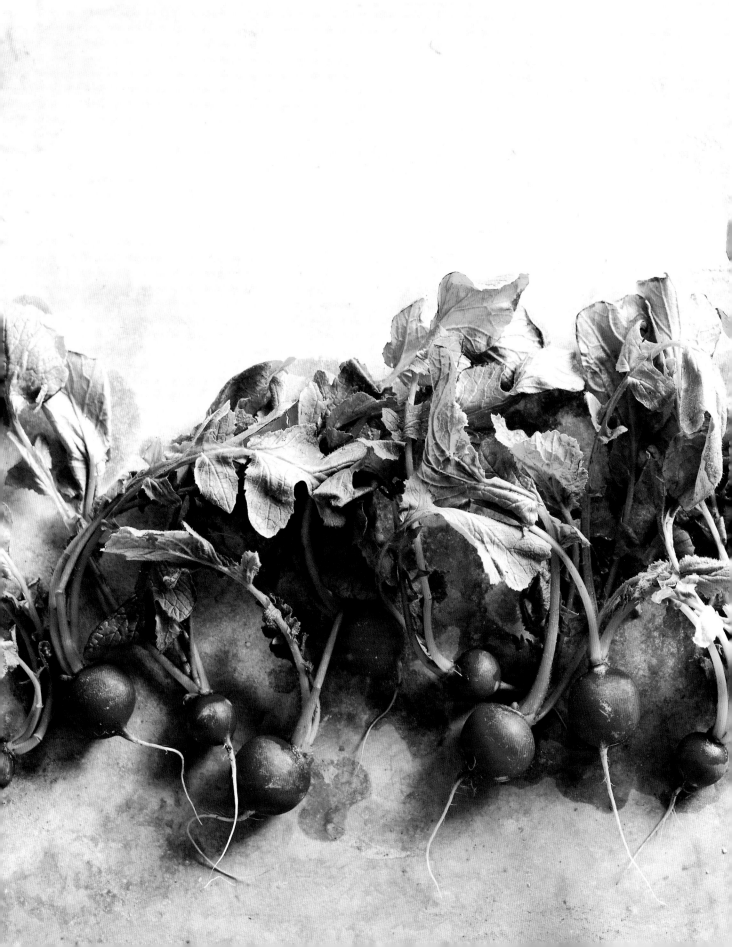

ACHIEVING AND MAINTAINING A HEALTHY BODY WEIGHT

ALL OVER THE WORLD, IN BOTH DEVELOPED AND developing nations, people are growing taller and getting heavier. In Australia, for example, we have been growing just over 1 cm taller per decade since 1899 — an amazing achievement brought about at least in part by improved nutrition and public health. Over the past few decades, however, we have been gaining more weight than we have been growing in height, leading to increasing rates of overweight and obesity.

In Australia, the most recent national health survey found that over two-thirds (69.7%) of all men, more than half (55.7%) of all women and one-quarter (25.1%) of all children are overweight or obese. The most recent survey in the UK also found that 67.9% of men, 59.4% of women and 28% of children are overweight or obese.

Of course, the flip side of these gloomy statistics is that nearly four out of 10 adults and three out of four children are not overweight or obese, and these people probably want to remain within the healthy weight range for their height, without gaining the average 0.5 to 1 kg each year that most of us manage to achieve.

How do you shape up?

The most commonly used tool for assessing a person's relative weight is known as the Body Mass Index (BMI). Your BMI can be calculated by dividing your weight in kilograms by your height in metres squared, or:

$$BMI = \frac{Weight\ (kg)}{Height\ (m) \times Height\ (m)}$$

For example, if you weigh 80 kg and are 1.75 m tall, your BMI would be 80 ÷ (1.75 x 1.75) = 26.1 kg/m^2.

Once you have calculated your BMI, you can see which category you fall into:

WEIGHT CATEGORY (FOR ADULTS)	BMI
Underweight	Less than 18.5 kg/m^2
Normal weight	Between 18.5 and 24.9 kg/m^2
Overweight	Between 25 and 29.9 kg/m^2
Obese	More than 30 kg/m^2

While being overweight or obese, as defined by the BMI, has been found to increase the average person's risk of developing a number of common conditions like type 2 diabetes, heart disease, stroke and some cancers, our BMI does not always give us the complete picture. For example, athletes can have a high BMI, but few are overweight, let alone obese. The reason is their larger than average lean body mass (for example, muscle) is beneficial to health, not a risk. On the other hand, some people may have a BMI less than 25 kg/m², but still be at risk of developing these health conditions because they have a smaller than average lean body mass and a larger proportion of body fat. Therefore, the BMI is not always a perfect tool for determining whether you are normal weight, overweight or obese. To help overcome some of these limitations of the BMI, it is also important to consider where you carry your weight. This is where waist measurement comes in.

Measuring your waist is easier than calculating your BMI. First, take a tape measure and carefully run it evenly around your stomach, halfway between the top of your hip bones and the bottom of your rib cage, and record the result (ask a family member or friend to help out for best results). Next, find out what category you are in, according to the table below.

If you are very tall, or very short, measures of body weight and circumference are probably not ideal for you. The ratio of your waist circumference relative to your height (waist-to-height ratio or WHR) is a relatively new way of finding out whether you are at risk of developing conditions like type 2 diabetes and heart disease. It is not affected by extremes in height or your ethnic background and it is very easy to measure and calculate. Simply measure your waist circumference and height in centimetres (or inches if you prefer) and divide the value for your waist by the value for your height. If the value is greater than 0.5 then you are at increased risk of developing pre-diabetes or type 2 diabetes.

$$WHR = \frac{\text{Waist circumference (cm)}}{\text{Height (cm)}}$$

For example, if your waist circumference is 91 cm and you are 175 cm tall, your waist to height ratio would be 91 ÷ 175 = 0.52, so you are at increased risk.

GENDER	HEALTHY	OVERWEIGHT	OBESE
Men	up to 94 cm for people of European descent and up to 90 cm for people of other ethnic backgrounds	94 to 102 cm	102 cm and over
Women	up to 80 cm	80 to 88 cm	88 cm and over

Rather than going on the latest fad diet, it's far more prudent to make small incremental changes, slowly swapping healthier foods and drinks for the regular varieties you have been consuming.

Losing weight and keeping it off

In order to successfully lose weight and also keep it off, you basically have to eat and drink less, and move more. Making small, sustainable changes to your lifestyle that don't dramatically change the types of food you like, don't cost too much and don't take up too much valuable time are the best ways to go.

Your weight loss goals should be realistic. Losing between 0.5 and 1 kg a week is optimal, because at this rate you will be losing mostly body fat, not lean muscle tissue. This means you won't be slowing down your metabolic rate, or inadvertently making yourself fatter (proportionately). Losing between 0.5 and 1 kg is equivalent to losing one to two 500 g tubs of margarine — it's a lot of fat when you think about it!

As far as how much you should lose, that depends on your starting weight. For people with pre-diabetes, losing 7.5% of current body weight can prevent more than five out of 10 people from developing type 2 diabetes. If you already have diabetes and you are overweight, losing 5 to 10% of your body weight can help improve your diabetes management, and as a consequence it can reduce your risk of developing the common complications of diabetes.

So what does 5 to 10% of your body weight mean in real terms? For an 80 kg person, this would mean losing 4 to 8 kg.

Successful long-term weight loss

We all know that losing weight and then maintaining that weight loss is not easy — particularly if we take the perspective of going on 'a diet' for a short period of time to lose a few kilograms. Whatever the latest fad weight loss diet is — be it low carbohydrate, low sugar, low fructose, wheat free or low fat — chances are that you won't be able to maintain it in the long run due to overwhelming feelings of hunger, boredom or inconvenience, or the fact that it clashes with your deeply ingrained familial and cultural habits. Even if you have the willpower to dramatically change your eating habits in the short term and achieve some weight loss, fad diets are not a recipe for long-term success for most people.

Many fad weight loss diets are also detrimental to long-term health. The underlying secret to most fad diets is over-restriction of kilojoules to facilitate rapid weight loss. This is usually achieved by almost completely avoiding one ingredient or food group. Unfortunately, the typical physical response to these semi-starvation diets is to use less of your body fat stores as a fuel in order to conserve energy, and to use your muscle and organs as energy sources instead. This may end up making you have more fat relative to your muscles, slowing down your metabolic rate. When you inevitably go back to your old eating habits, you put on more fat because of your slower metabolic rate, so you decide you need to go on a diet again — it can set you up for a vicious cycle of 'yoyo' dieting. The bottom line is that in the long run, 'diets' don't work.

Rather than going on the latest fad diet, it's far more prudent to make small incremental changes to your diet, slowly swapping healthier foods and drinks over the course of a few months for the regular varieties you have been consuming for many, many years. Or in other words, 'Swap it, don't stop it'! This approach works best in the long run — prohibition has never proven successful.

EAT AND DRINK LESS KILOJOULES

The average man consumes about 10 000 kJ each day in Australia and 9000 kJ each day in the UK, and the average woman consumes about 7500 kJ in Australia and 7000 kJ in the UK. To lose around 0.5 kg of body fat per week, you need to eat about 2000 kJ a day less. Therefore, for a typical man, this means eating and drinking a total of around 7000 to 8000 kJ a day, and 5000 to 5500 kJ a day for a typical woman.

Thinking about it from a slightly different perspective, most people need to consume about one-quarter less kilojoules each day than what they currently consume. Keep that figure in mind when you are purchasing, preparing and eating foods — it is a simple concept that can come in very handy.

One way to achieve this kilojoule reduction is to swap higher kilojoule versions of your favourite foods with lower kilojoule varieties as mentioned previously, or alternatively to eat and drink smaller portions of these foods.

EAT A MODERATELY HIGH PROTEIN, LOW-GI DIET

The Diogenes study from Europe recently proved that a moderately high protein, low-GI diet is the best for longer-term weight management. Fortunately, it is very easy for people to eat according to this pattern. We already eat a moderately high-protein diet — so there's no need for most of us to eat extra meat or dairy. Simply stick with what you are eating now and cut back on excess alcohol, fatty foods and refined carbohydrates (starches and sugars) instead. Most of us eat too many high-GI carbohydrates, so making sure that most of the carbohydrate foods you eat are low GI is also an important swap to make.

WATCH WHAT YOU DRINK

Fruit juices, regular soft drinks and alcohol are all concentrated sources of kilojoules and in order to lose weight you should limit them as much as possible. Diet versions of most soft drinks and cordials are commonly available and, other than water, are the best choice for those trying to lose weight — swap these for your regular varieties. As a community, we seem to overlook the fact that alcoholic drinks like wine and beer provide many more kilojoules per serve than soft drinks, and contribute more kilojoules to the typical person's diet. If you are trying to lose weight, drink no more than one standard alcoholic drink a day if you are a woman and no more than two standard alcoholic drinks if you are a man.

MOVE MORE

For general health, we need to do at least 30 minutes of physical activity each day. To lose body fat, we need to do around an hour a day. There are many different types of planned and incidental activities that are suitable choices.

Walking is one of the favourites for people of all ages. Research has shown that simply walking between 2 and 5 km (or between 2400 and 6400 steps) more than what you currently do each day will have benefits for the average person with diabetes. You can use your smartphone or a pedometer to measure how many kilometres or steps you walk each day during a typical week and then add the 2400 to 6400 steps to that figure to work out your goal.

BE CAREFUL WITH MEDICATION IF YOU ALREADY HAVE DIABETES

Reducing your food intake, particularly carbohydrates, increasing physical activity levels, and ultimately losing weight may lead to a reduction in the amount of diabetes medication or insulin that you need to take. Discuss your plans with your doctor or diabetes educator and check in regularly to ensure you are taking the optimal amount.

GET SOME PERSONALISED ADVICE

Members of your diabetes management team like your registered or accredited dietitian, exercise specialist (physiotherapist or exercise physiologist) and diabetes educator can provide you with more personalised advice that will make losing weight much easier and more sustainable. These experts are available at most local hospitals and community centres, and in private clinics.

THE BOTTOM LINE

If you want to lose weight, don't go on a diet — plan to make changes to your lifestyle that will help you lose weight at a safe rate and also keep it off for the long term.

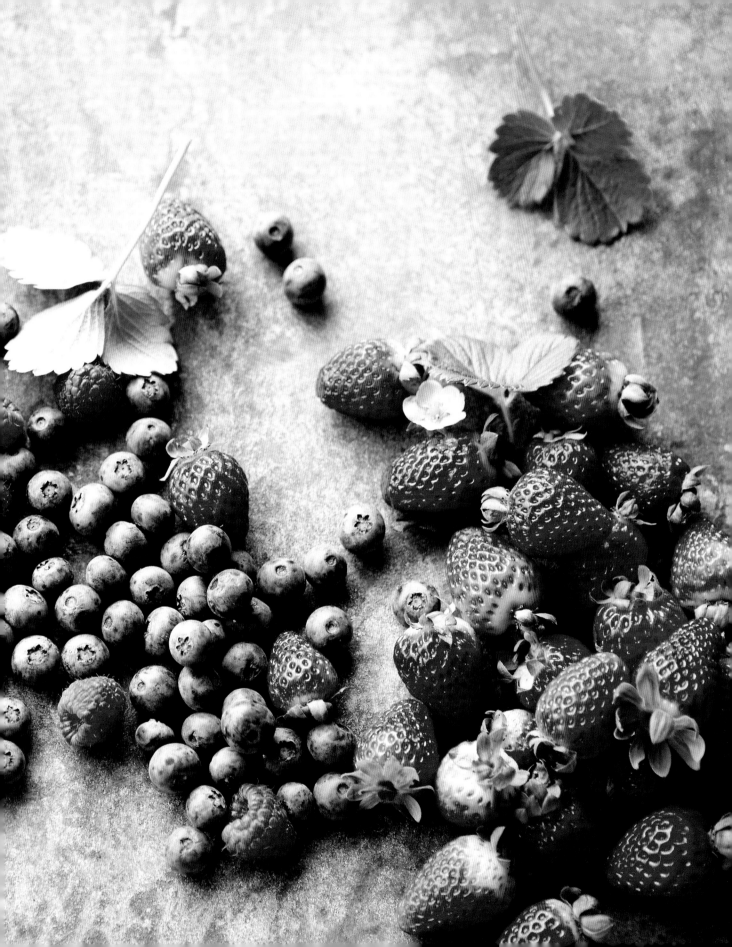

WE ALL KNOW THAT BEING PHYSICALLY ACTIVE, buying fresh ingredients and cooking healthy home-made foods is the best recipe for long-term weight loss and maintenance. However, despite our best efforts, we don't always have the time or inclination to prepare our own meals, or sometimes we really do need to lose weight fast — if we need to have urgent surgery, for example. Are there any safe and effective alternatives for people with diabetes or those at risk?

The answer is a qualified 'yes'. Very low energy diets are a special kind of meal replacement that can be used under certain circumstances for short periods of time to help you to lose weight rapidly. Alternatively, meal replacement programs can provide you with healthy kilojoule-controlled pre-prepared meals that will help you to lose weight safely and effectively, albeit at a slower rate than very low energy diets.

Very low energy diets

There is evidence that a special kind of weight loss diet known as a very low energy diet (VLED) can help people to lose more weight than regular healthy diets in the short term (less than a year). This can be very useful if you need to lose weight rapidly for surgery, or to help alleviate another acute health problem, such as severe joint or back pain. However, there is little evidence that VLEDs are any better for medium-to long-term (1 to 5 year) weight management.

VLEDs are diets that provide less than 3300 kJ a day. They are designed to produce rapid weight loss while preserving lean body mass (muscles and organs). This is accomplished by providing relatively large amounts of protein, typically 70 to 100 g a day. The protein is usually from milk-, soy- or egg-based powders, which are mixed with water or skim milk and consumed as a 'shake'. Depending on the formulation, typical VLEDs provide between 45 and 90 g of carbohydrate a day and between 2 and 20 g of fat a day, and provide 100% of the recommended daily allowance for most vitamins and minerals. On top of this you need to drink 2 litres of non-caloric fluids (for example, water, black tea, black coffee or diet soft drinks), and eat preferably 2 cups of non-starchy vegetables (for example, most vegetables other than potatoes, sweet potatoes, yams, pumpkin/winter squash, corn, peas, carrots, beetroot/beets, and parsnip) each day.

VLEDs are generally only recommended for people with diabetes who have a body mass index greater than 30 kg/m². Because they can be relatively low in carbohydrate, your diabetes medications or insulin may need to be reduced to prevent hypos. Also,

Very low energy diets (VLEDs) are generally only recommended for people with diabetes who have a body mass index greater than 30 kg/m². It is very important that you discuss using a VLED with your doctor and dietitian before commencing.

the high protein content of VLEDs may put a strain on your kidneys, which can be a serious problem if you have kidney disease. For these reasons, it is very important that you discuss using a VLED with your doctor and dietitian before commencing.

Once they were only found behind the counter of pharmacies, but now some VLED formulas can be found in the health food aisle in supermarkets. Originally they only came in the form of shakes, but now there are alternatives like bars, soups and even desserts. Typically, a person will follow a VLED exclusively for a 3-month period, and then they will progressively reduce the use of the shakes and replace them with regular healthy meals over the course of a few weeks to months.

Meal replacement programs

Designed for people who don't like shakes or other similar kinds of meal replacement formulas, most meal replacement programs provide between 4200 and 6300 kJ a day. They are nutritionally complete (provide enough protein, fat, carbohydrate, vitamins and minerals for the typical adult) and consist of main meals, soups and desserts. Due to the higher

kilojoule content, they do not promote as rapid weight loss in the short term as VLEDs. However, the evidence suggests that they are as effective as VLEDs in the medium term.

As meal replacement programs may contain different amounts of carbohydrate and protein to your regular meals, it is also wise to consult your doctor and dietitian before commencing.

THE BOTTOM LINE

Neither VLEDs nor meal replacement programs teach you how to buy and prepare healthy and appetising meals yourself. They are designed for individuals — not families — and if you are the main cook in your household, you will most likely have to prepare regular meals for the rest of the family, which may be inconvenient and costly, and can also create tension.

However, many people with diabetes or pre-diabetes can use VLEDs or meal replacement programs to safely lose weight in the short term. If you have sound medical reasons for needing to lose weight rapidly, you can discuss with your doctor and dietitian whether these options are suitable for you.

DIETARY SUPPLEMENTS

IT'S RARE TO SEE A CASE OF TRUE VITAMIN OR mineral deficiency in people with diabetes. However, high blood glucose levels, one of the characteristic symptoms of diabetes, may lead to the individual needing to urinate more, which in turn means that some B-group vitamins, vitamin C and certain minerals may be lost. In cases of people with a long history of undiagnosed or poorly managed diabetes, this could lead to borderline deficiencies. Also, some people taking Metformin may develop a vitamin B_{12} deficiency, so a B_{12} supplement may be necessary for them.

When average blood glucose levels are kept within the recommended range through healthy eating, physical activity and appropriate insulin or medication, vitamin and mineral requirements are essentially the same for people with diabetes as they are for those without.

Vitamin or mineral deficiencies arising from other diseases or conditions should be diagnosed and evaluated by your doctor or another qualified health professional. They will provide treatment on an individual basis, which may include vitamin or mineral supplementation.

Some vitamins and minerals can be toxic when they are consumed in amounts that greatly exceed the Recommended Dietary Intake (RDI) — the amount of each nutrient that the average adult requires each day (see Table 2, opposite page). Also, the excessive consumption of one vitamin or mineral may cause a deficiency of another vitamin or mineral. For example, large doses of vitamin C can decrease the absorption of vitamin B_{12}, and large doses of zinc can interfere with the absorption of copper.

It can be dangerous to self-treat a vitamin or mineral deficiency without knowing the underlying cause. However, those seeking some 'nutrition insurance' can use the following checklist:

1) Are your blood glucose levels kept within the recommended range most of the time? If not, consult your diabetes health care team to help you improve your blood glucose management.
2) Do you have clear symptoms of deficiency (see Table 2)? You should check with your doctor before going any further.
3) Try to correct any true deficiency by improving your food intake first.
4) If you decide to use dietary supplements, try to choose those that provide amounts that are as close to the RDI as possible (see Table 2).
5) Make sure that the supplement does not provide any more than 10 times the RDI of any nutrient.
6) Take supplements for the shortest time necessary.

Table 2: Vitamin and mineral requirements for adults*

VITAMIN/MINERAL	RDI	FOOD SOURCE	SYMPTOMS OF DEFICIENCY	SYMPTOMS OF TOXICITY
Vitamin A	M 900 µg F 700 µg	Liver, margarine, eggs, dark green leafy vegetables, yellow and orange fruits and vegetables	Night blindness; dry skin; xerophthalmia (dry eyes); increased risk of infections and cancer.	Headaches; bone and joint pain; dry, itchy skin
Vitamin B_1 (Thiamine)	M 1.2 mg F 1.1 mg	Whole grains, meat, legumes, Vegemite	Fatigue; depression; reduced mental functioning; muscle cramps; nausea; heart enlargement; beri-beri	Anorexia; fatigue; irritability; insomnia
Vitamin B_2 (Riboflavin)	M 1.3 mg F 1.1 mg	Meat, dairy foods, whole grains, Vegemite	Red, swollen, cracked mouth and tongue; greasy, scaly skin on face	Non-toxic
Vitamin B_3 (Niacin)	M 16 mg F 14 mg	Meat, fish, poultry, peanuts, whole grains, Vegemite	Pellagra (dermatitis, diarrhoea and dementia); weakness; poor appetite; sore mouth	Flushing; headaches; gastrointestinal disturbances
Vitamin B_6	M 1.7 mg F 1.5 mg	Meat, fish, eggs, whole grains, Vegemite	Weakness; poor appetite; dermatitis; sore mouth; increased infections; anaemia	Nerve damage
Folate	M 400 µg F 400 µg	Liver, green leafy vegetables, legumes, whole grains, fortified cereals	Anaemia	Non-toxic, but large doses can mask vitamin B_{12} deficiency
Vitamin B_{12}	M 2.4 µg F 2.4 µg	Meat, fish, eggs, dairy products	Pernicious anaemia; fatigue; light-headedness; headache and irritability	Non-toxic
Vitamin C	M 45 mg F 45 mg	Fruits and vegetables	Scurvy (bleeding gums, easy bruising, dry skin); increased infections; increased risk of cancer, heart and blood vessel disease	Diarrhoea; nausea; kidney stones; rebound scurvy when megadoses are stopped
Vitamin D	M 10 µg F 10 µg	Cod liver oil, table margarines and spreads, salmon, herring, sardines, eggs, some milks and dairy foods (fortification is voluntary)	Demineralisation of bones (osteoporosis and osteomalacia); increased infections; poor skin	Excess calcium in the blood (hypercalcaemia), which can cause poor appetite, nausea and vomiting; weakness, frequent urination and kidney problems may occur
Vitamin E	M 10 mg F 7 mg	Vegetable oils, whole grains, nuts and seeds, green leafy vegetables	May increase risk of heart and blood vessel disease and cancer	Non-toxic
Calcium	M 1000 mg F 1300 mg	Dairy foods, nuts and seeds, green leafy vegetables	Osteoporosis, high blood pressure	Nausea; vomiting; kidney, heart and muscle damage
Iron	M 8 mg F 8 mg	Meat, fish, poultry, whole grains, green leafy vegetables	Weakness; fatigue; increased infections; anaemia	Damage to the gastrointestinal tract; liver damage
Zinc	M 14 mg F 8 mg	Meat, fish, legumes, nuts	Skin problems; immune deficiency	Vomiting; diarrhoea; copper deficiency

KEY: M = RDI for adult men aged 51 to 70 years, F = RDI for adult women aged 51 to 70 years, µg = micrograms, mg = milligrams

*Source: Nutrient Reference Values for Australia and New Zealand including Recommended Dietary Intakes. Commonwealth Department of Health and Ageing, Australia, and Ministry of Health, New Zealand. National Health and Medical Research Council. 2006

HEALTHY EATING ON A BUDGET

THE COST OF LIVING CONTINUES TO RISE, AND having enough money to enjoy healthy foods and drinks is an issue that concerns many people. It is almost folklore that eating healthily costs you more money. For most people, this need not be the case. Healthy eating on a budget simply requires a bit of careful planning and some appropriate food storage and preparation facilities at home. Here are some practical tips.

GETTING ORGANISED

- Plan what meals you're going to eat and when. Make sure you vary your meals. You will get bored and lose motivation if you don't experiment with different ingredients and recipes. To help you do this, we have provided 70 tempting recipes in *Reversing Diabetes* for you to enjoy with your family and friends.
- Determine how much money you have for food.
- Check newspaper advertisements, store flyers or on-line catalogues for weekly specials, and take advantage of special offers.
- Make a detailed shopping list before you head to the shops.

SHOPPING

- Buy quality home-brand versions of core foods, e.g. bread, pasta, rice and tinned tomatoes.
- Home-brand products are often nutritionally equal to the more expensive brand name foods.
- Buy a smaller amount of the premium-quality lean meats rather than more of the cheaper cuts or processed meats (including sausages).
- Buy fruits and vegetables that are in season, and if possible, go to a local growers' market where prices are lower — but make sure you're getting good-quality produce.
- Go to the market with a friend or group of friends. As well as being more fun, bulk buying is generally a lot cheaper.
- Frozen vegetables or tinned fruit and vegetables in light or natural juice, or water, are good alternatives to fresh — they're available out of season and are usually as nutritious.
- Use unit pricing in supermarkets, which allows you to compare prices of items across different sizes and also across different items.

STORING

Stock up on the following items when they are on special:

- rice, pasta and lentils
- tinned beans, chickpeas and lentils
- tinned fish, e.g. salmon, tuna, sardines and mackerel

- frozen vegetables
- tinned vegetables, e.g. tomatoes and corn kernels
- UHT reduced-fat or skim milk and desserts
  (e.g. reduced-fat custard)
- packet and tinned soups (limit 'cream of' varieties
  because these are usually higher in kilojoules and
  saturated fat)
- tinned fruit in light or natural juice or water
- dried fruit, e.g. apricots, dates and prunes
- dried herbs and spices, curry powder, vinegars,
  tomato sauce (ketchup), soy sauce and stock
  (bouillon) cubes.

COOKING

- Beans, peas and lentils are great value-for-money
  sources of protein — use them to bulk out stews,
  curries and casseroles.
- Use a small amount of grated strong cheese
  (e.g. parmesan) for flavour instead of larger
  amounts of less flavoursome cheese.
- If you're a couple, prepare recipes for four or six
  people so you can use the leftovers for a quick
  meal the following night or freeze the leftovers
  for another night.

MANAGING LEFTOVERS

To minimise the risk of food poisoning, it is important
that you handle all leftovers carefully.

- Cooked leftovers should be cooled as quickly as
  possible and then stored in the fridge or freezer
  (within 1½ hours).
- Eat leftovers within 2 days (if you haven't frozen
  them).
- Eat dishes that contain rice within 1 day.
- Ensure that food is covered before storing it in
  the fridge.
- When reheating food, always make sure it is piping
  hot all the way through — be especially careful if
  using the microwave.
- Do not reheat dishes more than once.

READING
FOOD LABELS

IN AUSTRALIA, NEW ZEALAND (NZ), THE UK and many other parts of the world, packaged foods provide nutrition information including ingredients lists, nutrition information panels and nutrition content claims such as 'high fibre' or 'low fat', to help people to work out if the food suits their individual nutritional requirements.

Ingredients lists

The ingredients list is a useful tool for people who want to know exactly what is in their foods and drinks. Ingredients are declared in descending order of weight. If sugar, for example, is the first ingredient on the list, you know that the food or drink contains a relatively large quantity of sugar, and if it is last on the list, it contains relatively little.

In Australia, NZ and the European Union (EU), food companies are also required to list the percentage of key characterising ingredients in the ingredients list. For example, strawberry yoghurt must state in the ingredients list the percentage of strawberries that are actually in the yoghurt.

Ingredients must be listed using either:
• the common name of the ingredient, or
• a name that describes the true nature of the ingredient, or, where applicable,
• a generic name that can be used to describe a range of similar ingredients (e.g. 'sugar' can describe white sugar, caster/superfine sugar, cube sugar, icing/confectioners' sugar, coffee sugar, coffee crystals or raw sugar).

Nutrition information panels

In many countries, including Australia and NZ, nutrition information panels are mandatory on nearly all packaged foods, whereas in the UK, EU and many countries they are not mandatory unless a food makes a nutrition content claim. However, recent estimates from the EU indicate that 85% of foods and drinks provide some form of nutrition information, and companies are transitioning over to a new mandatory system by December 2016 as part of a recent agreement within the EU.

Around the globe, nutrition information panels provide, as an absolute minimum, information about the amount of energy (kilojoules and/or calories), protein, fat and carbohydrate in 100 g or 100 ml of the food or drink. In most countries information panels must also include information on saturated fats, sugars and sodium. In the UK and other parts of the EU, salt is listed instead of sodium.

Nutrition information on food labels is regulated by government authorities in Australia, NZ and the UK.

In Australia and NZ, amounts of all nutrients must be listed in a 'serve' of food or drink as well as in 100 g, whereas in the UK information per serve or portion is voluntary. The serving sizes themselves are not regulated by government, and they may not always be the same as what you would normally eat or drink yourself, but the information can be useful as a general guide.

Nutrition claims

There is a wide range of nutrition content claims like 'low fat', 'reduced fat', 'low sugar', 'no added sugar', 'high fibre', 'low salt', 'no added salt' and so on that are allowed on the labels of food. Perhaps unsurprisingly, these claims tend to accentuate the positive and downplay the negative ingredients, and while they may be technically correct (they are defined by law in Australia, NZ and the EU), they can be misleading. Most confectionery, for example, is low in fat, but most is also devoid of any nutrients other than carbohydrate (usually highly refined sugars like glucose or sucrose), so the information is arguably little more than a thinly disguised marketing ploy. On the whole, it's best to look at the ingredients list and nutrition information panel rather than the nutrition claims.

Some of the more common nutrition claims are explained below to help you fully understand what they mean.

FAT

Low-fat foods are defined as those that contain no more fat than:
• 1.5 g per 100 ml in liquid foods, or
• 3 g per 100 g in solid foods.

Reduced-fat foods must contain at least 25% less fat than the amount contained in the same quantity of a similar reference food.

It is unnecessary to specifically look for low-fat or reduced-fat foods. The quality of the fats contained in the food is more important than the total quantity.

Foods low in saturated and trans fats are defined as those that contain no more than:
• 0.75 g per 100 ml in liquid foods, or
• 1.5 g per 100 g in solid food.

These figures are useful for lower-fat foods and drinks, but are not necessarily ideal for higher-fat varieties. A more useful measure for higher-fat foods is the saturated to unsaturated fat ratio. This information isn't provided directly in a food's nutrition information panel, but you can calculate it relatively easily.

Usually, the nutrition panel only lists the amount of total fat and saturated fat, but if a fat claim is made such as 'low fat' or 'reduced fat', the amount of trans fats, mono- and polyunsaturated fats are also listed. There are therefore two ways of working out the amount of unsaturated fat in foods. Either:
• subtract the amount of saturated fat from total fat, or
• add the amount of mono-unsaturated fat and polyunsaturated fat together.

You can use this information to calculate the saturated to unsaturated fat ratio — simply divide the amount of saturated fat by the total amount of unsaturated fat. If the result is less than 0.5, then the food has an optimal saturated to unsaturated fat ratio that will help reduce your total and LDL cholesterol levels.

Salt and sodium conversions

To convert salt to sodium, divide the salt value by 2.5 and then multiply it by 1000. To convert sodium to salt, multiply the sodium value by 2.5 and then divide it by 1000.

CARBOHYDRATE

Perhaps surprisingly, given the popularity of low-carbohydrate diets and the number of 'low-carb' claims on foods and drinks, there are no specific food regulations that define 'low carbohydrate' claims on food labels. There are regulations for 'reduced carbohydrate' and sugars, however.

Foods promoted as reduced carbohydrate must provide at least 25% less carbohydrate than that found in the same quantity of a reference food.

Foods promoted as low in sugars must contain no more than:
• 2.5 g per 100 ml in liquid foods; or
• 5 g per 100 g in solid foods.

Perhaps surprisingly, given the popularity of low-carbohydrate diets and the number of 'low-carb' claims on foods and drinks, there are no specific food regulations that define 'low carbohydrate' claims on food labels.

Foods promoted as being reduced in sugars must contain at least 25% less than the same quantity of a similar reference food.

Notice that both the claims about sugars relate to total sugars — not added sugar. The sugars content of a food or drink does not determine how it will affect your blood glucose levels, so choosing foods or drinks low or reduced in sugars will not necessarily mean that they will help you manage your diabetes or pre-diabetes more effectively.

FIBRE

In Australia, NZ and the UK, fibre is not a mandatory component of the nutrition information panel. Only when a claim is made about fibre, sugars or starch, must the fibre content be listed.

Because fibre is seen as a 'positive' nutrient, manufacturers like to advise us if their foods contain appreciable amounts to draw our attention to the potential benefits of consuming their product.
- To claim a food is a 'good source' of fibre, a serving of the food must contain at least 4 g of dietary fibre.
- To claim a food is an 'excellent source' of fibre, a serve must contain at least 7 g of dietary fibre.

- To claim a food has 'increased' fibre, the reference food must contain at least 2 g of dietary fibre per serving, and the food must contain at least 25% more dietary fibre than the same quantity of the reference food.

SODIUM

Foods that are promoted as being low in sodium must contain no more than 120 mg per 100 ml in solid or liquid foods.

Reduced-sodium foods must contain at least 25% less sodium than the same quantity of a similar reference food.

No-added-salt foods must contain no added sodium compound including no added salt, and the ingredients of the food must contain no added sodium compound including no added salt.

Front of pack labelling

In Australia and NZ, the Health Star Rating is a voluntary front-of-pack labelling scheme that shows how packaged foods rate out of five stars — with five out of five stars being the highest rated and 0.5 out of five stars being the lowest. This rating is calculated using a complex formula that takes into account the amount of energy (kJ), saturated fat, total sugars, sodium, fibre, protein, and the percentage of fruits, vegetables, nuts and legumes in 100 g/100 ml of a food or beverage. In addition to the star rating, the amount of energy, saturated fat, total sugars, sodium and fibre may also be provided on the front of the pack, with an optional statement indicating whether the food is high or low in that particular nutrient.

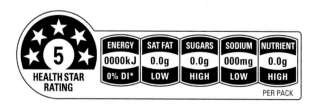

Similarly, in the UK, there is a voluntary front-of-pack labelling scheme for packaged foods that is a colour-coded version of the daily intake guide for energy, plus fat, saturated fat, sugars and salt in 100 g/100 ml of a food or drink. The energy content can appear by itself, or with the other four nutrients. For any particular nutrient, a colour rating can be incorporated, grading the food from low (green) to high (red), for that particular nutrient.

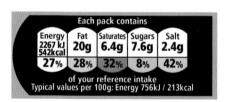

Both these systems are useful guides for the general population to help improve packaged food choices. They are not specifically designed to help people prevent or manage diabetes, however. Neither the Australian nor UK models incorporate total carbohydrate, for example, so people who have diabetes still need to look at the nutrition information panel in order to assess the amount of this vital nutrient in a food or beverage.

Nutrition information
Balsamic chicken with
potato and fennel bake
Recipe page 170

Nutrition	Per serve
Energy (kJ)	1500
Protein (g)	38
Carbohydrate (g)	24
Starches (g)	12
Sugars (g)	12
Exchanges	1.5
Portions	2.5
GI	Low
GL	Low
Protein:carbohydrate ratio	1.58
Fat (g)	9
Saturated fat (g)	3
Unsaturated fat (g)	6
Saturated:unsaturated ratio	0.5
Fibre (g)	6
Sodium (mg)	175
Potassium (mg)	1610
Sodium:potassium ratio	0.11
Gluten free?	Yes

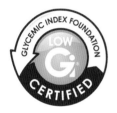

GI SYMBOL

Foods that carry the GI symbol have had their glycaemic index tested at an accredited laboratory and they must also meet strict nutrient criteria for kilojoules, saturated fat and sodium, as well as fibre and calcium where appropriate. The nutrient criteria are consistent with international dietary guidelines and were developed in consultation with experts from Diabetes Australia and the University of Sydney.

Nutrition information accompanying the recipes in this book

Even though every recipe in *Reversing Diabetes* has been designed to meet the general requirements of all people with diabetes and pre-diabetes, we recognise the fact that everyone is truly an individual and therefore personal requirements may vary. In order to help you decide if a particular recipe is right for you, each one contains comprehensive nutrition information so that you can make up your own mind. Please use the following information about energy, protein, fat, saturated fat, carbohydrate, sodium, potassium and gluten content to assist you in your decision making.

ENERGY

The average estimated daily requirement for adult Australians and New Zealanders is 8700 kJ per day, and for the EU it is 8400 kJ. Most people eat three main meals and some people choose to eat snacks, so if you divide the figure by three or four, depending on your eating pattern, you can see that the average person's main meal could provide between 2100 and 2900 kJ, and if you snack, you could divide the fourth 2100 kJ by the number of snacks you eat.

However, we don't all eat the same size meal for breakfast, lunch and dinner. Depending on the amount of time you have and your personal preferences, one meal is usually larger than the others. These figures are averages, and we are all different, so only use them as a general guide.

PROTEIN

The recommended dietary intake for protein is 64 g a day for an average man and 46 g a day for a woman. Taking the same approach as we have taken for energy, an average man would need 16 to 22 g of protein at each meal, and an average woman would need 12 to 16 g at each meal as a general guide.

FAT

There isn't a recommended dietary intake for fat because the kind of fat you eat is more important than the amount. However, fat is a concentrated source of energy (kilojoules). As a guide, choose dishes that contain no more than 25 g of total fat in a single serve to help limit your kilojoule intake.

SATURATED FAT

For optimal health, you should aim to have twice as much unsaturated fat as you have saturated fat, or in other words, the ratio of saturated to unsaturated fats should be less than 0.5. Of course, you don't have to achieve this aim at every single meal — it's the long-term average that counts.

CARBOHYDRATE

Like fat, there isn't a recommended dietary intake for carbohydrate. Carbohydrate has the most profound impact on blood glucose and insulin levels, however, so some diabetes organisations recommend that most adults have no more than 63 g at main meals and 33 g for snacks. Many people count grams of carbohydrate, or use 15 g carbohydrate exchanges or 10 g portions to help match their insulin or blood glucose lowering medication to their requirements. We have included both for your convenience. A 15 g exchange includes foods with 12–18 g of carbohydrate and a 10 g portion 7.6–12.5 g of carbohydrate.

One way of assessing carbohydrate quality is by looking at the amount of starch and sugars in a food or drink. We have also included both of these for your convenience.

Glycaemic index (GI) and glycaemic load (GL) are the best indicators of carbohydrate quality for people with diabetes, since they predict how foods affect your blood glucose levels. Ideally, most meals on most days will be low GI and low GL, but it is all right to have the occasional medium-GI or medium-GL meal or snack. Adults consuming 8700 kJ each day should aim to have less than 100 units of GL, or 25 to 33 units at main meals and 8 to 11 at snacks, depending on your eating pattern.

For optimal feelings of fullness, it's recommended that the protein to carbohydrate ratio of a meal is at

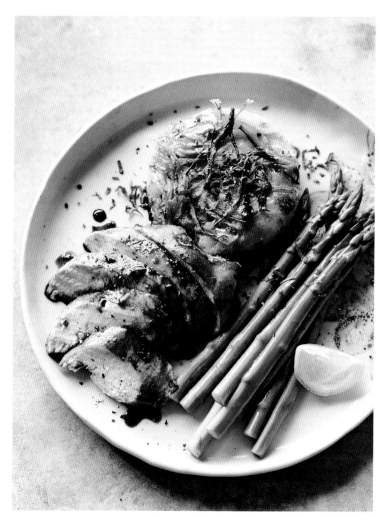

Balsamic chicken with potato and fennel bake is a low-GL, gluten-free meal.
Recipe page 170

SODIUM

The WHO recommends that we consume less than 2000 mg of sodium a day. Taking the same approach as we have for energy and protein, an average adult should aim to consume less than 500 mg of sodium at each meal and 165 mg for snacks. Some diabetes organisations recommend you aim to eat less than the upper limit and suggest choosing main meals that contain less than 450 mg of sodium and small meals, snacks or desserts that contain less than 150 mg.

POTASSIUM

The estimated adequate intake for potassium is 3800 mg a day for men and 2800 mg for women. Taking the same approach as for sodium, an average man would need 950 mg of potassium at each meal, and an average woman would need 700 mg at each meal as a general guide.

From a cardiovascular disease risk perspective, the ratio of sodium to potassium is arguably more important than the total amount of either mineral. Ideally, you will have at least as much potassium as you have sodium in a meal to balance it out, so the ratio should be no greater than 1.

GLUTEN FREE

We have indicated which recipes are gluten free. This assumes that all of the ingredients that you use are gluten-free varieties.

For optimal feelings of fullness, it's recommended that the protein to carbohydrate ratio of a meal is at least one to two. This means eating at least 1 g of protein for every 2 g of carbohydrate. Meals that have a protein to carbohydrate ratio greater than 0.5 are the best choices.

MEAL PLAN: *Week One**

	MONDAY	TUESDAY	WEDNESDAY
BREAKFAST	• 35 g (1¼ oz/¼ cup) natural muesli • 125 ml (4 fl oz/½ cup) reduced-fat milk or alternative • 1 lady finger banana 1445 kJ; 58 g Carbs	• 70 g (2½ oz/⅔ cup) raw rolled (porridge) oats • 125 ml (4 fl oz/½ cup) reduced-fat milk or alternative • 2 teaspoons wildflower honey 1465 kJ; 58 g Carbs	• 2 slices sourdough toast • 220 g (7¾ oz) tinned salt-reduced baked beans 1290 kJ; 50 g Carbs
LUNCH	• Roasted beetroot, lentil and goat's cheese salad (page 138)	• Rosemary lamb and vegetable kebabs with lemon cracked wheat (page 169)	• Chicken poached in fragrant Asian broth (page 110)
SNACK	• Pumpkin, polenta and herb muffin (page 92)	• 200 g (7 oz/¾ cup) reduced-fat plain yoghurt • ½ lady finger banana	• 1 piece fresh fruit
DINNER	• Spiced vegetable pilaf with lamb fillets (page 180)	• Spelt spaghetti with ratatouille (page 125)	• Pan-fried river trout with sautéed potatoes (page 131)
DESSERT	• 200 g (7 oz/¾ cup) reduced-fat plain yoghurt • Fresh strawberries	• Berry sponge cake with honeyed ricotta (page 213)	• Apple crumble (page 210)

THURSDAY	FRIDAY	SATURDAY	SUNDAY
• 70 g (2½ oz/1 cup) bran-based breakfast cereal • 125 ml (4 fl oz/½ cup) reduced-fat milk or alternative • ½ lady finger banana 1410 kJ; 48 g Carbs	• 175 g (6 oz/1 cup) seasonal fruit salad • 200 g (7 oz/¾ cup) reduced-fat plain yoghurt • 1 slice toasted fruit bread with 1 teaspoon margarine 1350 kJ; 47 g Carbs	• Buckwheat pancakes with berries (page 209)	• 2 slices sourdough toast • 2 small poached eggs • Grilled (broiled) mushrooms, tomato and asparagus 1800 kJ; 40 g Carbs
• Spanish tortilla pies (page 115)	• Turkey and sage burgers with onion and fennel relish (page 132)	• Spiced cauliflower and lentil soup (page 109)	• Minestrone with barley and croutons (page 112)
• 200 g (7 oz/¾ cup) reduced-fat plain yoghurt • ½ lady finger banana	• 1 piece fresh fruit	• Cinnamon oat biscuit (page 206)	• Fruit and nut energy slice (page 96)
• Lamb seekh kebabs with minted yoghurt (page 178)	• Beef and bean nachos (page 161)	• Chipotle barbecued chicken with sweet potato wedges (page 189)	• Poached chicken with roasted pumpkin and herb dressing (page 165)
• Almond chia pudding with caramelised pineapple (page 217)	• 200 g (7 oz/¾ cup) reduced-fat plain yoghurt	• Baked chocolate egg custard (page 218)	• French apple tart (page 214)

MEAL PLAN: *Week Two**

	MONDAY	TUESDAY	WEDNESDAY
BREAKFAST	• 70 g (2½ oz/1 cup) bran-based breakfast cereal • 125 ml (4 fl oz/½ cup) reduced-fat milk or alternative • ½ lady finger banana 1410 kJ; 48 g Carbs	• 175 g (6 oz/1 cup) seasonal fruit salad • 200 g (7 oz/¾ cup) reduced-fat plain yoghurt • 1 slice toasted fruit bread with 1 teaspoon margarine 1350 kJ; 47 g Carbs	• 70 g (2½ oz/⅔ cup) raw rolled (porridge) oats • 125 ml (4 fl oz/½ cup) reduced-fat milk or alternative • 2 teaspoons wildflower honey 1465 kJ; 58 g Carbs
LUNCH	• Chilli chicken and coriander quesadillas (page 104) • 1 piece fresh fruit	• Spiced pork and water chestnut dumpling soup (page 106)	• Chicken and quinoa patties (page 105)
SNACK	• 1 slice Rye and caraway bread (page 88)	• 1 piece fresh fruit	• Pumpkin and barley scone (page 95)
DINNER	• Teriyaki salmon with soba noodles and pickled vegetables (page 126)	• Tarragon chicken and beans (page 183)	• Dukkah-crusted lamb cutlets with jewelled couscous (page 129)
DESSERT	• 200 g (7 oz/¾ cup) reduced-fat plain yoghurt • ½ lady finger banana	• Almond chia pudding with caramelised pineapple (page 217)	• Cinnamon oat biscuit (page 206)

THURSDAY	FRIDAY	SATURDAY	SUNDAY
• 2 slices sourdough toast • 2 scrambled eggs • 125 ml (4 fl oz/½ cup) 100% orange juice 1880 kJ; 37 g Carbs	• 35 g (1¼ oz/¼ cup) natural muesli • 125 ml (4 fl oz/½ cup) reduced-fat milk or alternative • 1 lady finger banana 1445 kJ; 58 g Carbs	• 2 slices sourdough toast • 2 slices grilled (broiled) short cut (lean back) bacon • Grilled (broiled) mushrooms, tomato and asparagus • 125 ml (4 fl oz/½ cup) 100% orange juice 1595 kJ; 39 g Carbs	• 2 slices sourdough toast • 2 small poached eggs • 220 g (7¾ oz) tinned salt-reduced baked beans 2300 kJ; 59 g Carbs
• Spiced cauliflower and lentil soup (page 109)	• Pasta with capsicum and rocket (page 150)	• Minestrone with barley and croutons (page 112)	• Spiced pepper quail with herb quinoa (page 194)
• 1 piece fresh fruit	• 200 g (7 oz/¾ cup) reduced-fat plain yoghurt	• Broad bean and ricotta dip with crudités (page 82)	• Spiced vegetable crisps (page 87)
• Lamb vindaloo (page 196)	• Tomato, mozzarella and olive quinoa pizza (page 149)	• Pulled pork with black bean salsa and fennel slaw (page 190)	• Pearl barley, leek and mushroom risotto (page 155)
• Baked chocolate egg custard (page 218)	• 1 piece fresh fruit	• Apple crumble (page 210)	• Berry sponge cake with honeyed ricotta (page 213)

Part Two
RECIPES

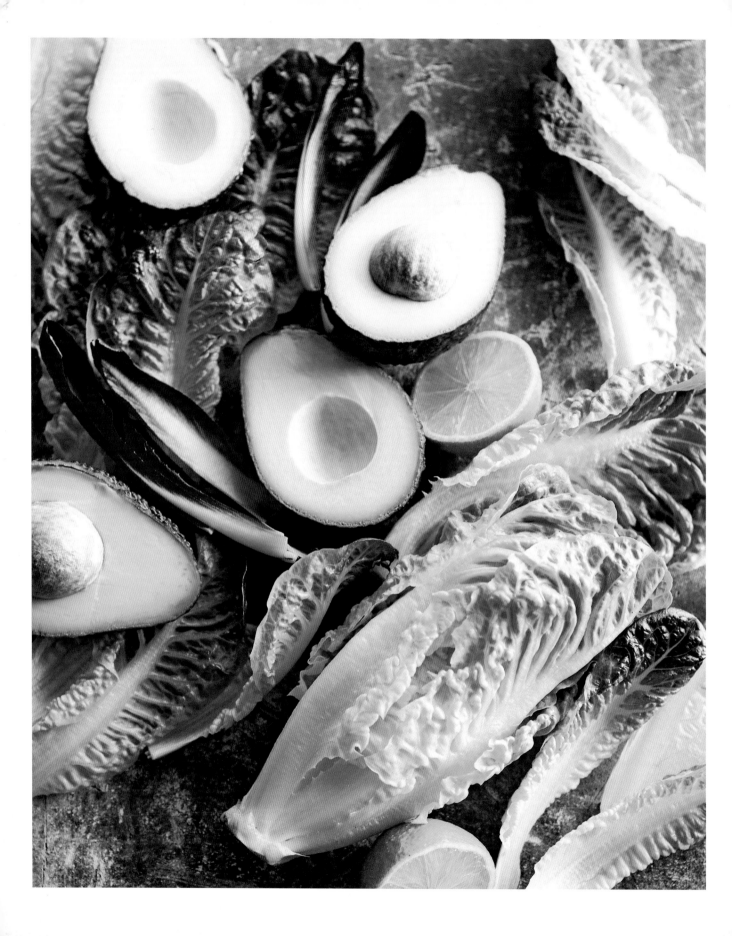

Chapter One

SNACKS

BROAD BEAN *and* RICOTTA DIP *with* CRUDITÉS

Broad beans (also known as fava beans) are a versatile legume with a high amount of dietary fibre and folate. They are also a good source of low-fat protein.

Ingredients

500 g (1 lb 2 oz) frozen broad beans, thawed

250 g (9 oz) extra light (1% fat) smooth ricotta cheese

2 spring onions (scallions), chopped

1 small handful mint leaves, plus extra sprigs to serve

2 teaspoons grated lemon zest

2 tablespoons lemon juice

150 g (5½ oz) baby carrots

100 g (3½ oz) radishes, trimmed

2 celery stalks, sliced on the diagonal

1 red capsicum (pepper), cut into thin wedges

1 Lebanese (short) cucumber, cut into thin wedges

Method

1 Add the broad beans to a saucepan of boiling water and cook for 5 minutes. Drain and refresh under cold running water, then slip off the skins.

2 Put the broad beans, ricotta, spring onions, mint leaves, lemon zest and lemon juice in the bowl of a food processor and purée until smooth. Season with freshly ground black pepper.

3 Serve the dip topped with mint sprigs, with the vegetables for dipping.

Serves 4
Preparation 20 minutes
Cooking 5 minutes

Nutrition	Per serve
Energy (kJ)	550
Protein (g)	14
Carbohydrate (g)	9
Starches (g)	2
Sugars (g)	7
Exchanges	0.5
Portions	1
GI	Low
GL	Low
Protein:carbohydrate ratio	1.56
Fat (g)	1.5
Saturated fat (g)	0.4
Unsaturated fat (g)	1.1
Saturated:unsaturated ratio	0.36
Fibre (g)	12
Sodium (mg)	210
Potassium (mg)	655
Sodium:potassium ratio	0.32
Gluten free?	Yes

notes

Substitute broad beans with other tinned varieties of beans, such as cannellini beans or chickpeas. Rinse and drain them before use. If you prefer a little heat, add a chopped fresh chilli when puréeing the dip.

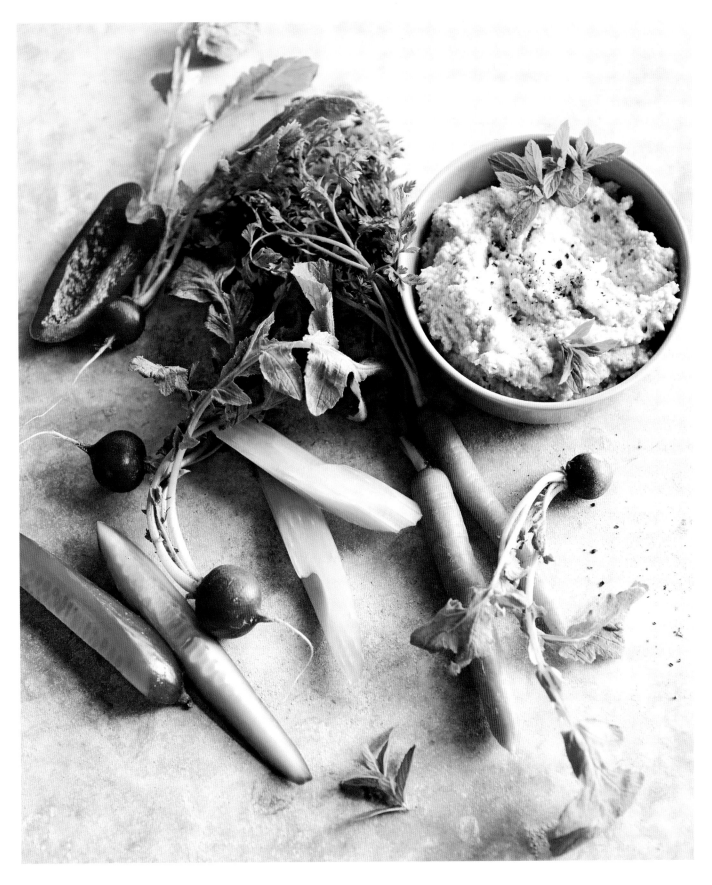

ROASTED TOMATO *and* CAPSICUM RELISH

Roasting capsicums brings out their natural sweetness. This healthy relish makes a good accompaniment to sandwiches and barbecued meats, or add a handful of basil leaves and toss it through hot pasta.

Ingredients

10 ripe roma (plum) tomatoes, halved

2 tablespoons balsamic vinegar

1 garlic bulb, halved crossways

2 large red capsicums (peppers), halved

Method

1 Preheat the oven to 180°C (350°F). Line two baking trays with baking paper. Arrange the tomatoes, cut side up, on one tray. Drizzle with the vinegar and season with freshly ground black pepper. Wrap the garlic in foil and add to the tray. Put the capsicums, cut side down, on the other tray.

2 Put the trays in the oven with the capsicums on the top shelf and the tomatoes and garlic on the lower shelf. Cook for 1 hour or until the tomatoes have softened and the capsicums start to blacken.

3 Wrap the capsicums in foil and set aside to sweat for 10 minutes. When cool enough to handle, peel away the skins and roughly chop the flesh.

4 Squeeze the garlic from the skin and add it to a food processor with the tomatoes and any cooking juices. Blend for 10 seconds or until the mixture is just combined and still lumpy. Transfer to a bowl and stir in the chopped capsicums.

Makes 1 litre (35 fl oz/4 cups)
Preparation 10 minutes +
10 minutes cooling
Cooking 1 hour

Nutrition	Per cup
Energy (kJ)	240
Protein (g)	3
Carbohydrate (g)	6
Starches (g)	1
Sugars (g)	5
Exchanges	0.5
Portions	0.5
GI	Low
GL	Low
Protein:carbohydrate ratio	0.5
Fat (g)	1
Saturated fat (g)	0.1
Unsaturated fat (g)	0.9
Saturated:unsaturated ratio	0.11
Fibre (g)	5
Sodium (mg)	11
Potassium (mg)	470
Sodium:potassium ratio	0.02
Gluten free?	Yes

note

Store the relish in sterilised jars in the refrigerator for up to 2 weeks.

ROCKET *and* BASIL PESTO

This vibrant pesto is low in carbohydrate and high in healthy unsaturated fats. Add a few tablespoons to pasta dishes, use it as a spread for bread or spoon it on top of roasted vegetables.

Ingredients

120 g (4¼ oz/2¾ cups) baby rocket (arugula)
150 g (5½ oz/2 bunches) basil leaves
2 tablespoons pine nuts
1 tablespoon finely grated parmesan cheese
60 ml (2 fl oz/¼ cup) lemon juice
60 ml (2 fl oz/¼ cup) extra virgin olive oil

Method

1 Wash and pat dry the rocket and basil leaves.

2 Put the rocket, basil, pine nuts and parmesan in the bowl of a food processor. Chop until combined.

3 Add the lemon juice and olive oil, and blend until the pesto is smooth.

Makes 375 ml (13 fl oz/1½ cups)
Preparation 10 minutes
Cooking Nil

Nutrition	Per cup
Energy (kJ)	1700
Protein (g)	6.5
Carbohydrate (g)	5
Starches (g)	1
Sugars (g)	4
Exchanges	0
Portions	0.5
GI	Low
GL	Low
Protein:carbohydrate ratio	1.33
Fat (g)	40
Saturated fat (g)	5
Unsaturated fat (g)	35
Saturated:unsaturated ratio	0.14
Fibre (g)	5
Sodium (mg)	80
Potassium (mg)	670
Sodium:potassium ratio	0.12
Gluten free?	Yes

notes

Store the pesto in sterilised jars in the refrigerator for up to 2 weeks.
Substitute the basil with mint to make a sauce to serve with lamb dishes.

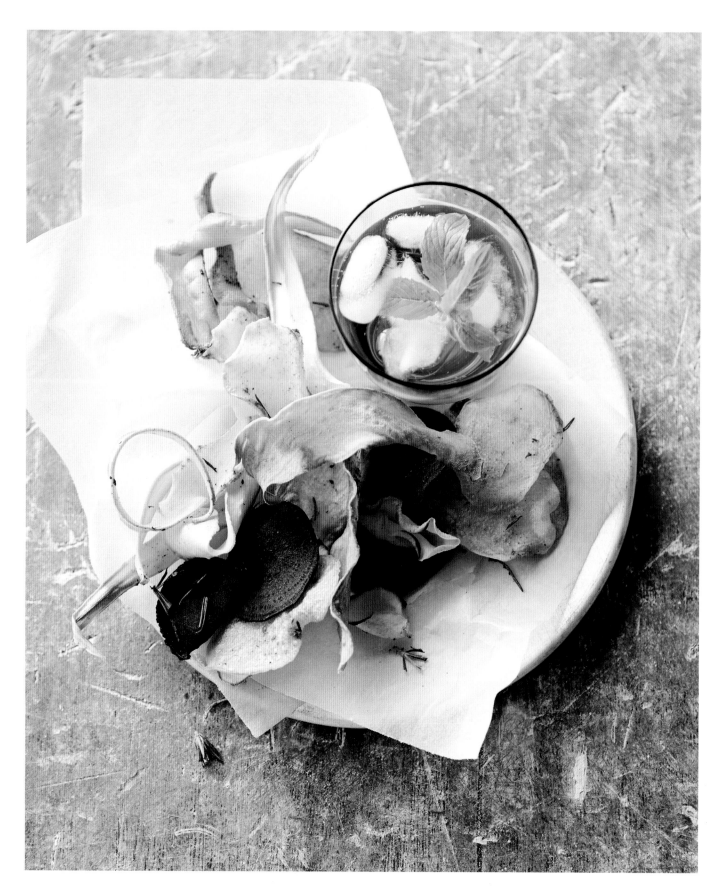

SPICED VEGETABLE CRISPS

Unlike commercial varieties, these oven-baked crisps are very low in fat, and high in fibre and potassium. They don't contain the saturated fat of deep-fried chips or the high GI of crisps made using regular potatoes.

Ingredients

1 small (200 g/7 oz) orange sweet potato
1 x 80 g (2¾ oz) swede (rutabaga)
1 x 100 g (3½ oz) parsnip
1 x 150 g (5½ oz) beetroot (beet)
1 x 150 g (5½ oz) lower-GI potato, such as Carisma
1 x 100 g (3½ oz) carrot
olive oil spray
1 tablespoon rosemary leaves, chopped
2 teaspoons Cajun spice mix

Method

1 Preheat the oven to 190°C (375°F). Place two wire racks on two baking trays.

2 Use a mandolin or large sharp knife to cut the peeled vegetables into paper-thin slices. Pat dry with paper towel. Arrange the vegetable slices in a single layer on the wire racks. Lightly spray with olive oil and sprinkle with the chopped rosemary and Cajun spice mix.

3 Bake the vegetables for 45 minutes, swapping the trays over halfway, or until golden and crisp. Cool the crisps for 15 minutes before serving.

Serves 4 as a snack
Preparation 20 minutes
Cooking 45 minutes

Nutrition	Per serve
Energy (kJ)	450
Protein (g)	3
Carbohydrate (g)	18
Starches (g)	5
Sugars (g)	13
Exchanges	1
Portions	2
GI	Medium
GL	Low
Protein:carbohydrate ratio	0.17
Fat (g)	1
Saturated fat (g)	0
Unsaturated fat (g)	1
Saturated:unsaturated ratio	N/A
Fibre (g)	6
Sodium (mg)	45
Potassium (mg)	620
Sodium:potassium ratio	0.07
Gluten free?	Yes

notes

The crisps are best eaten on the day they are made. Try cooking some kale in the same way for a healthy snack.

RYE *and* CARAWAY BREAD

This loaf is made using rye flour, and toasts well for a breakfast meal. It is a good source of fibre, as well as being low in sodium and high in potassium.

Ingredients

2 teaspoons instant dried yeast
1 teaspoon light brown sugar
240 g (8½ oz/1½ cups) rye flour
225 g (8 oz/1½ cups) stone-ground plain (all-purpose) flour, plus 2 tablespoons for kneading
25 g (1 oz/¼ cup) rolled (porridge) oats
2 tablespoons chia seeds
2 tablespoons caraway seeds
1 tablespoon linseeds (flaxseeds)
olive oil spray
1 teaspoon semolina

Method

1 Combine the yeast with the brown sugar and 375 ml (13 fl oz/1½ cups) tepid water in a bowl. Stir until the yeast has dissolved, then set aside for 10 minutes or until frothy.

2 Put the flours in a large bowl. Combine the oats and seeds in another bowl. Set aside a pinch of the oat mixture for sprinkling, add the remaining mixture to the flours and mix to combine. Make a well in the centre, then pour in the yeast mixture and stir until the dough comes together. Turn the dough out onto a lightly floured surface and knead for 8–10 minutes or until smooth and elastic. Return the dough to the lightly oiled bowl, cover with a clean tea towel (dish towel) and rest in a warm place for 1½ hours or until doubled in size.

3 Lightly spray a 9 x 19 cm (3½ x 7½ inch) loaf (bar) tin (base measurement) with olive oil and sprinkle with the semolina. Using your hands, knock back the dough to its original size. Knead the dough for 2–3 minutes, then roll into a log shape. Cut three diagonal slashes into the top of the log. Place in the prepared tin, sprinkle with the reserved oat and seed mixture, cover and set aside to rise for 45 minutes.

4 Preheat the oven to 200°C (400°F). Bake the bread for 35–40 minutes or until the top is golden and the loaf sounds hollow when tapped on the base. Transfer to a wire rack to cool before slicing.

Makes 1 loaf (16 slices)
Preparation 15 minutes + 2 hours 25 minutes resting and rising
Cooking 40 minutes

Nutrition	Per slice
Energy (kJ)	510
Protein (g)	4
Carbohydrate (g)	18
Starches (g)	17.5
Sugars (g)	0.5
Exchanges	1
Portions	2
GI	Medium
GL	Low
Protein:carbohydrate ratio	0.22
Fat (g)	2
Saturated fat (g)	0.3
Unsaturated fat (g)	1.7
Saturated:unsaturated ratio	0.18
Fibre (g)	4
Sodium (mg)	3
Potassium (mg)	135
Sodium:potassium ratio	0.02
Gluten free?	No

notes

Try adding different seeds, such as sunflower seeds or pepitas (pumpkin seeds). If you are toasting this bread, note that it will take a little longer to turn golden than other breads.

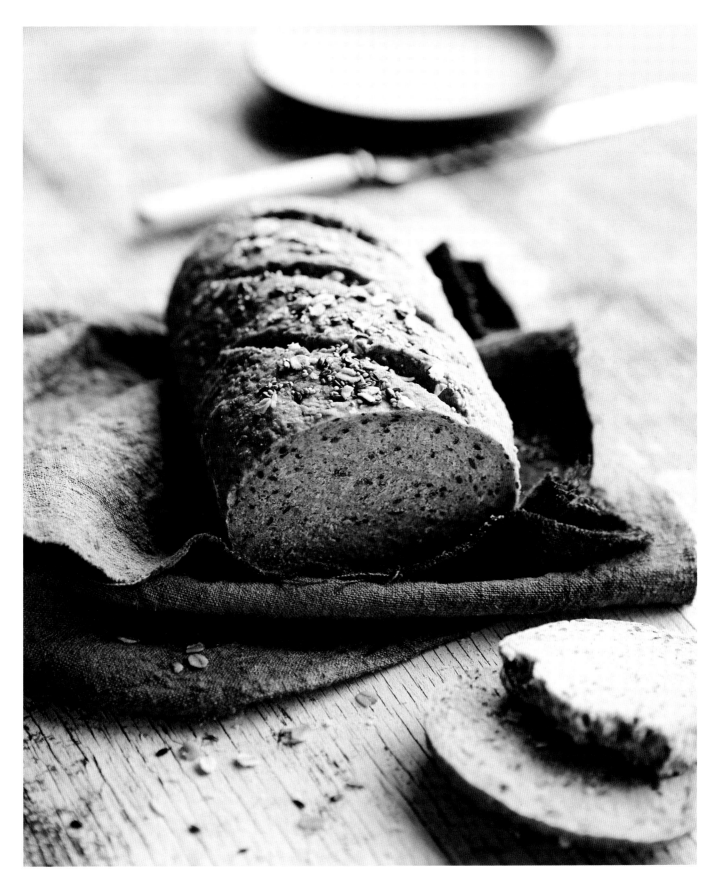

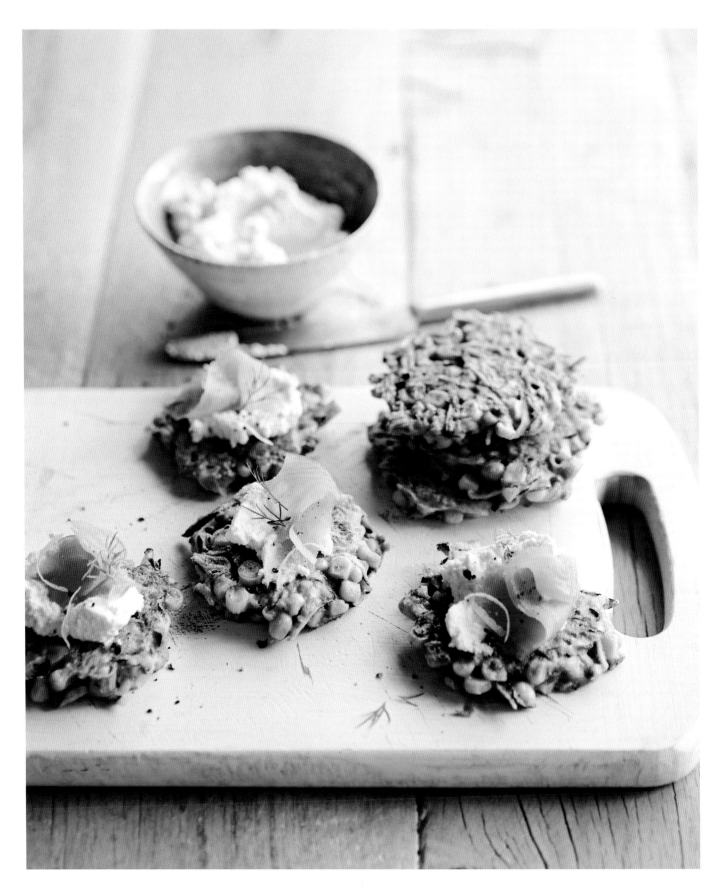

ZUCCHINI *and* CORN FRITTERS *with* SMOKED SALMON

Buckwheat flour is a gluten-free flour and an excellent source of fibre and micronutrients. It has a nutty taste and originates from the same plant species as rhubarb.

Ingredients

olive oil spray

1 corn cob, kernels removed

2 large (300 g/10½ oz) zucchini (courgettes), coarsely grated

2 spring onions (scallions), thinly sliced

35 g (1¼ oz/¼ cup) buckwheat flour

½ teaspoon smoked paprika

2 eggs, lightly whisked

2 tablespoons dill sprigs, chopped, plus extra to serve

250 g (9 oz) extra light (1% fat) smooth ricotta cheese

80 g (2¾ oz) smoked salmon, roughly chopped

finely grated lemon zest, to serve

Method

1 Spray a large non-stick frying pan with olive oil and heat over medium–high heat. Cook the corn kernels, stirring, for 3–4 minutes or until softened. Transfer to a large bowl to cool.

2 Add the zucchini, spring onions, buckwheat flour and paprika to the corn and stir until combined. Add the eggs and chopped dill, and mix until just combined. Season the batter with freshly ground black pepper.

3 Spray the same frying pan with olive oil and heat over medium heat. Using a heaped tablespoon of the batter for each fritter, cook the fritters in several batches for 2 minutes on each side or until golden. Transfer to a wire rack to cool.

4 To serve, top each fritter with a dollop of ricotta, some smoked salmon, extra dill, lemon zest and freshly ground black pepper.

Serves 4 (Makes 12)
Preparation 15 minutes
Cooking 20 minutes

Nutrition	Per serve
Energy (kJ)	800
Protein (g)	16
Carbohydrate (g)	16
Starches (g)	13
Sugars (g)	3
Exchanges	1
Portions	1.5
GI	Low
GL	Low
Protein:carbohydrate ratio	1
Fat (g)	6
Saturated fat (g)	1.5
Unsaturated fat (g)	4.5
Saturated:unsaturated ratio	0.33
Fibre (g)	4
Sodium (mg)	450
Potassium (mg)	590
Sodium:potassium ratio	0.76
Gluten free?	Yes

notes

Make a double batch of the fritters and freeze half. For an alternative to smoked salmon, use shredded, skinless poached chicken and use a little mashed avocado instead of the ricotta.

PUMPKIN, POLENTA *and* HERB MUFFINS

Polenta is made by grinding dried corn. When used in baking it gives a granular texture and a slight crunch.

Ingredients

400 g (14 oz) peeled pumpkin (winter squash), cut into 4 cm (1½ inch) pieces
canola oil spray
150 g (5½ oz/1 cup) wholemeal (whole-wheat) self-raising flour
75 g (2½ oz/½ cup) self-raising flour
180 g (6 oz/1 cup) instant polenta (cornmeal)
½ small red capsicum (pepper), finely chopped
1 tablespoon thyme leaves
2 tablespoons pepitas (pumpkin seeds)
250 ml (9 fl oz/1 cup) buttermilk
2 eggs, at room temperature, lightly whisked
2 tablespoons grapeseed oil

Method

1 Steam the pumpkin for 5–10 minutes or until soft. Mash with a fork until smooth, then set aside to cool.

2 Preheat the oven to 200°C (400°F). Lightly spray a 12-hole standard (80 ml/2½ fl oz/⅓ cup) muffin tin with canola oil.

3 Combine the flours, polenta, capsicum, thyme and half the pepitas in a large bowl. Make a well in the centre.

4 Whisk the buttermilk, eggs and grapeseed oil in a bowl until combined. Stir the mashed pumpkin through the egg mixture, then pour into the dry ingredients and gently stir until just combined.

5 Divide the batter among the muffin holes and scatter the remaining pepitas over the top. Bake for 20–25 minutes or until the muffins are golden. Transfer to a wire rack to cool.

Makes 12
Preparation 15 minutes + cooling
Cooking 35 minutes

Nutrition	Per muffin
Energy (kJ)	810
Protein (g)	7
Carbohydrate (g)	26
Starches (g)	23
Sugars (g)	3
Exchanges	1.5
Portions	2.5
GI	Medium
GL	Medium
Protein:carbohydrate ratio	0.27
Fat (g)	6
Saturated fat (g)	1
Unsaturated fat (g)	5
Saturated:unsaturated ratio	0.2
Fibre (g)	3
Sodium (mg)	150
Potassium (mg)	145
Sodium:potassium ratio	1.03
Gluten free?	No

note

Store the muffins in an airtight container for 3 to 4 days, or wrap them individually and freeze for up to 3 months.

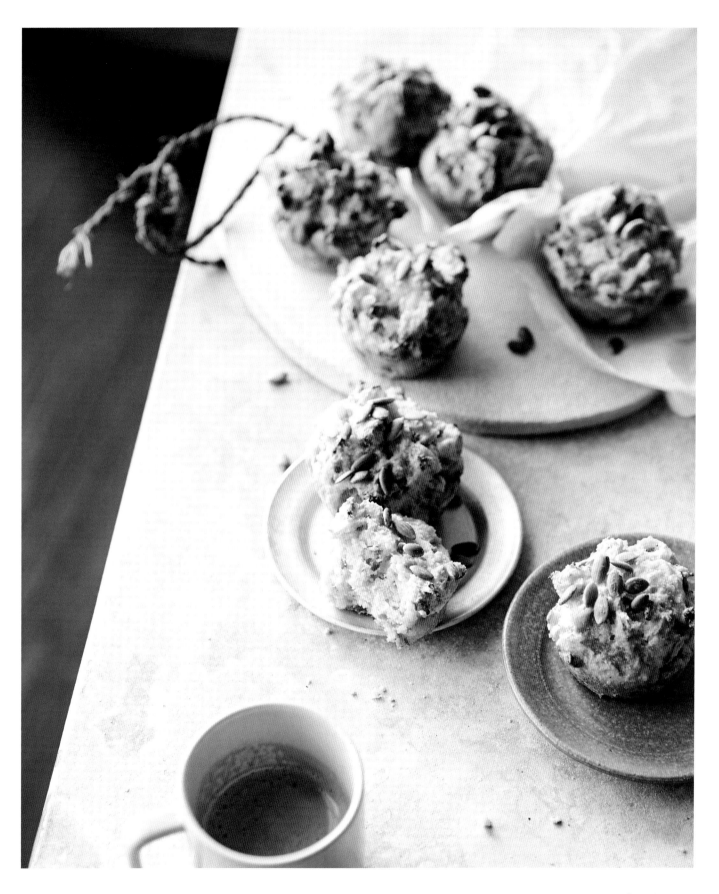

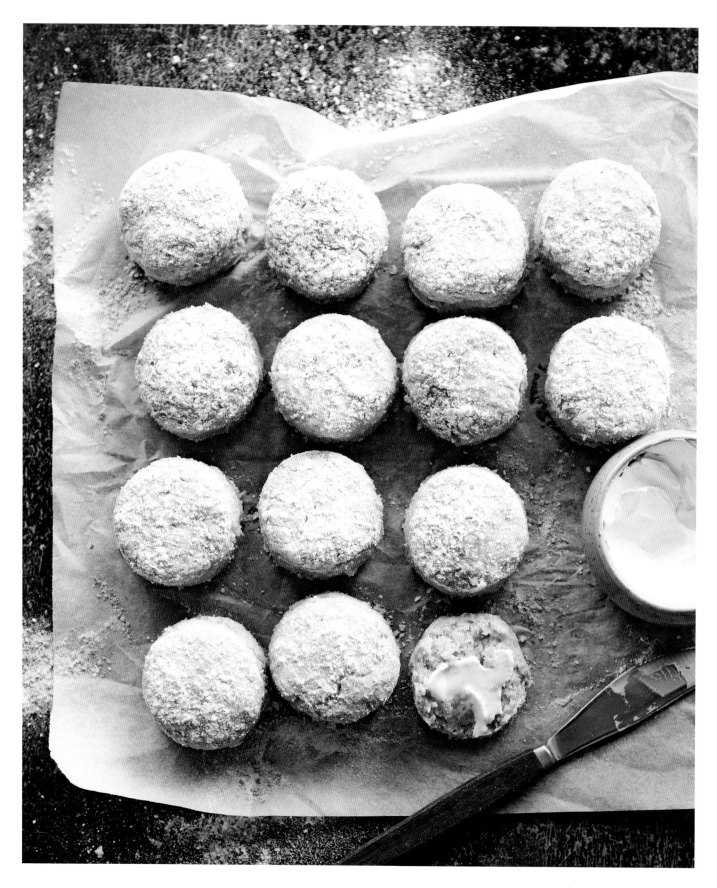

PUMPKIN *and* BARLEY SCONES

Barley flour is a non-wheat flour that is low in fat. It is made by milling the hulled barley grain.

Ingredients

400 g (14 oz) peeled butternut pumpkin (squash), roughly chopped

260 g (9¼ oz/2 cups) barley flour, plus 2 tablespoons for rolling and dusting

150 g (5½ oz/1 cup) wholemeal (whole-wheat) self-raising flour

1 teaspoon baking powder

½ teaspoon freshly grated nutmeg

40 g (1½ oz) reduced-fat canola spread, plus extra to serve (optional)

125 ml (4 fl oz/½ cup) buttermilk

Method

1 Preheat the oven to 200°C (400°F). Line a baking tray with baking paper.

2 Steam the pumpkin for 5–10 minutes or until soft. Mash with a fork until smooth, then set aside for 10 minutes to cool.

3 Combine the flours, baking powder and nutmeg in a bowl and sift together three times. Using your fingertips, rub the canola spread into the flour mixture until it resembles fine breadcrumbs. Add the pumpkin and buttermilk, and mix with a round-bladed knife using a cutting motion until the dough just comes together.

4 Turn the dough out onto a clean, lightly floured surface. Gently knead for 1 minute or until smooth. Use your fingertips to flatten the dough into a 2 cm (¾ inch) disc. Cut out 16 rounds using a 5 cm (2 inch) round cutter dipped in flour. Put the rounds on the prepared tray with the edges just touching and dust with a little extra barley flour.

5 Bake the scones for 12–15 minutes or until golden. Transfer to a wire rack and cover with a clean tea towel (dish towel) until ready to serve.

6 Serve the warm scones with canola spread (if using), allowing about 1 teaspoon for each scone.

Makes 16

Preparation 20 minutes + 10 minutes cooling

Cooking 25 minutes

Nutrition	Per scone
Energy (kJ)	470
Protein (g)	3
Carbohydrate (g)	18
Starches (g)	17
Sugars (g)	1
Exchanges	1
Portions	2
GI	Medium
GL	Low
Protein:carbohydrate ratio	0.17
Fat (g)	2.5
Saturated fat (g)	0.5
Unsaturated fat (g)	2
Saturated:unsaturated ratio	0.25
Fibre (g)	3
Sodium (mg)	115
Potassium (mg)	100
Sodium:potassium ratio	1.15
Gluten free?	No

notes

For pumpkin and herb scones, omit the nutmeg and add 2 tablespoons chopped mixed herbs. The scones will freeze well, wrapped individually and placed in an airtight container, for up to 3 months.

FRUIT *and* NUT ENERGY SLICE

Lupins are members of the legume family. Lupin flour is high in protein and dietary fibre, and low in fat. The low-GI carbohydrate in this slice will provide sustained energy.

Ingredients

canola oil spray

50 g (1¾ oz/½ cup) lupin flour

65 g (2¼ oz/½ cup) oat bran

50 g (1¾ oz/½ cup) rolled (porridge) oats

100 g (3½ oz) dried apricots, finely chopped

50 g (1¾ oz) dried figs, finely chopped

2 tablespoons unsweetened cacao powder

2 tablespoons roasted hazelnuts, chopped

2 tablespoons roasted almonds, chopped

1 tablespoon linseeds (flaxseeds)

2 tablespoons pepitas (pumpkin seeds)

2 eggs

2 tablespoons canola oil

65 g (2¼ oz/¼ cup) unsweetened apple purée

Method

1 Preheat the oven to 170°C (325°F). Lightly spray a 20 cm (8 inch) square cake tin with canola oil, then line the base and sides with baking paper, letting the paper extend over the sides.

2 Put the flour, oat bran, oats, apricots, figs, cacao, hazelnuts, almonds, linseeds and half the pepitas in a bowl and mix well.

3 Whisk the eggs, canola oil and apple purée in a small bowl, then pour into the dry ingredients and mix until combined.

4 Press the fruit and nut mixture into the prepared tin and scatter over the remaining pepitas. Bake for 25–30 minutes or until the slice is firm. Cool in the tin for 30 minutes before lifting out and cutting into 16 squares.

Makes 16 squares
Preparation 15 minutes
Cooking 30 minutes

Nutrition	Per square
Energy (kJ)	515
Protein (g)	5
Carbohydrate (g)	11
Starches (g)	6
Sugars (g)	5
Exchanges	0.5
Portions	1
GI	Low
GL	Low
Protein:carbohydrate ratio	0.45
Fat (g)	6
Saturated fat (g)	1
Unsaturated fat (g)	5
Saturated:unsaturated ratio	0.2
Fibre (g)	3
Sodium (mg)	30
Potassium (mg)	255
Sodium:potassium ratio	0.12
Gluten free?	No

note

Lupin flour is available from health food stores. It can be substituted with barley flour in this recipe.

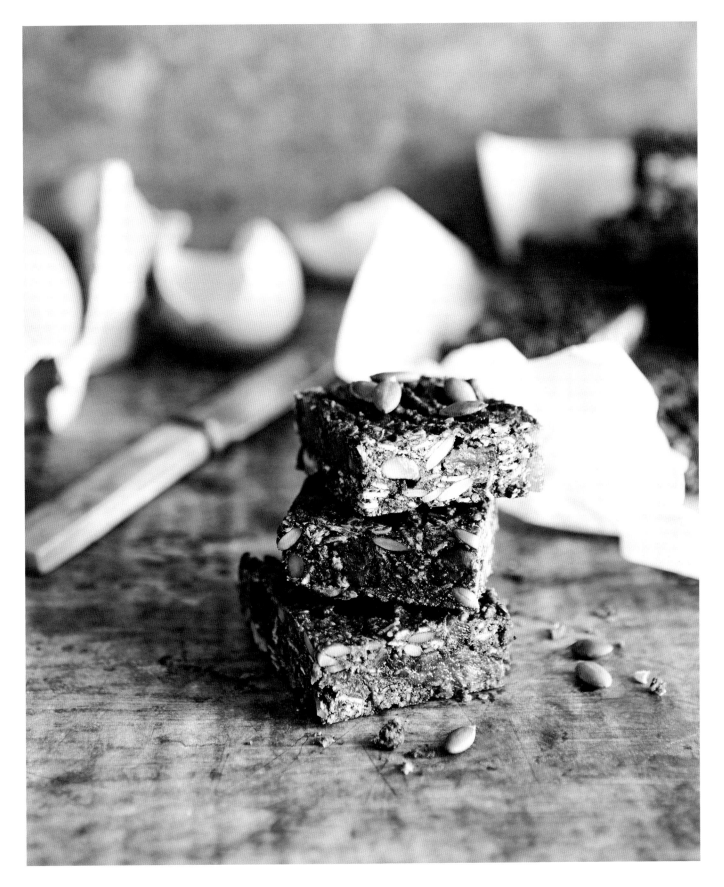

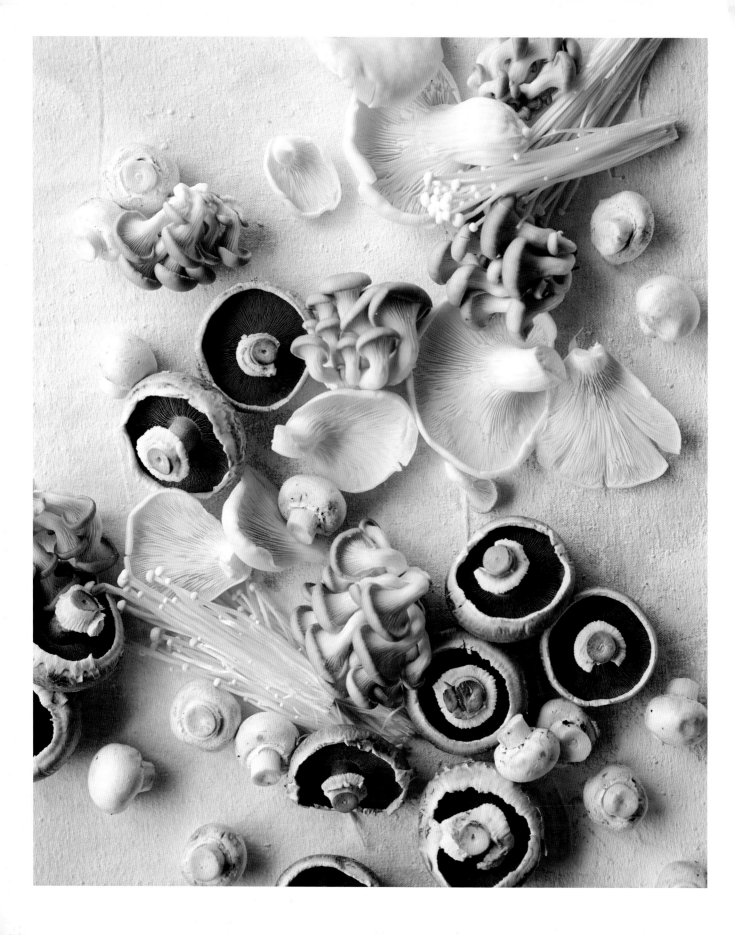

Chapter Two

SOUPS & LIGHT MEALS

BRUSCHETTA

Serve the bruschetta with some tinned tuna or sardines in springwater for extra protein. Any left-over tomatoes can be used in pasta dishes or tossed through salads.

Ingredients

12 x 10 g (¼ oz) slices wholegrain baguette
olive oil spray
1 garlic clove, halved
350 g (12 oz) mixed baby roma (plum) tomatoes
½ small red onion, thinly sliced
8 pitted black olives in oil, drained on paper towel, sliced
1 teaspoon extra virgin olive oil
2 tablespoons balsamic vinegar
1 small handful basil leaves

Method

1 Preheat the grill (broiler) to high. Put the baguette slices on a baking tray in a single layer and spray with olive oil. Turn and spray the other side. Cook under the grill for 2 minutes on each side or until golden. Rub the toasted baguette slices with the garlic.

2 Cut the tomatoes into halves or quarters and put them in a small bowl. Add the onion, olives, extra virgin olive oil and vinegar, and mix until combined.

3 To serve, divide the tomato mixture among the baguette slices and top with the basil leaves.

Serves 4
Preparation 15 minutes
Cooking 5 minutes

Nutrition	Per serve
Energy (kJ)	470
Protein (g)	3
Carbohydrate (g)	17
Starches (g)	12
Sugars (g)	5
Exchanges	1
Portions	1.5
GI	Medium
GL	Low
Protein:carbohydrate ratio	0.18
Fat (g)	2.5
Saturated fat (g)	0.3
Unsaturated fat (g)	2.2
Saturated:unsaturated ratio	0.14
Fibre (g)	3.2
Sodium (mg)	220
Potassium (mg)	295
Sodium:potassium ratio	0.75
Gluten free?	No

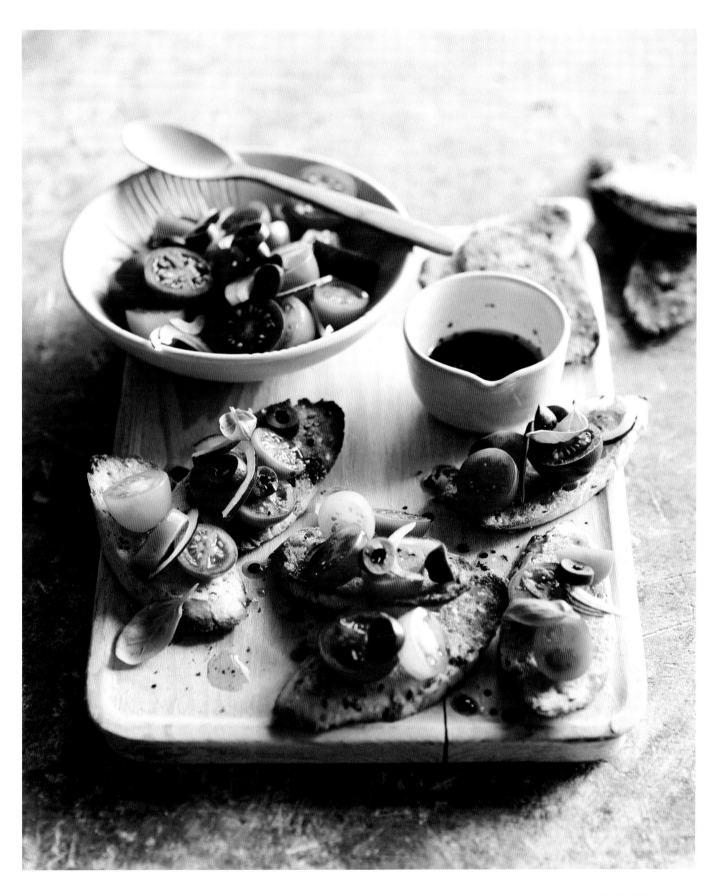

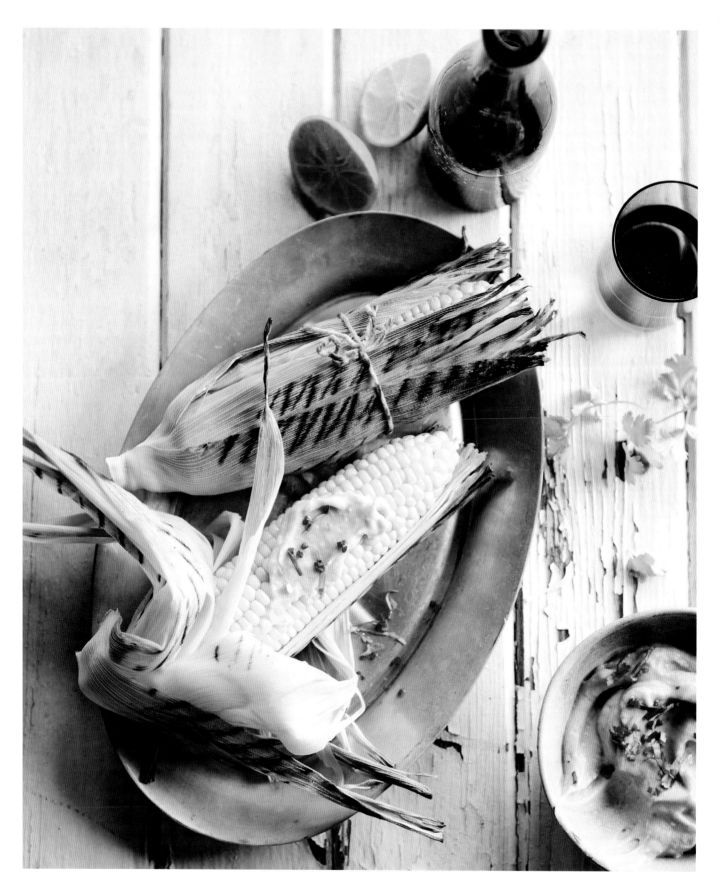

BARBECUED CORN *with* AVOCADO CREAM

The avocado cream can also be used as a creamy topping for jacket potatoes or as a spread for toast or sandwiches. It's full of healthy unsaturated fats, dietary fibre and potassium.

Ingredients

2 corn cobs, husks attached
1 long red chilli, finely chopped
lime cheeks, to serve

Avocado cream

1 small avocado
1 tablespoon lime juice
¼ teaspoon cayenne pepper
1 tablespoon coriander (cilantro) leaves, finely chopped

Method

1 Peel back the husks from the corn cobs, discard the silk and remove several of the inside husks, leaving a few outer husks to protect and steam the corn while it is cooking. Soak the corn cobs and two pieces of string in a large bowl of water for 15 minutes.

2 Meanwhile, to make the avocado cream, use a stick blender or small food processor to blend the avocado, lime juice and cayenne pepper until it reaches a smooth, spreadable consistency. Stir in the coriander and set aside until needed.

3 Preheat a barbecue or chargrill pan to medium-high. Drain the corn cobs, reseal the husks and secure with the wet string. Cook the corn, turning occasionally, for 15–20 minutes or until tender.

4 Peel back the husks and spread the corn with the avocado cream. Sprinkle with the chilli and serve with lime cheeks.

Serves 2
Preparation 5 minutes +
15 minutes soaking
Cooking 20 minutes

Nutrition	Per serve
Energy (kJ)	1790
Protein (g)	9
Carbohydrate (g)	27
Starches (g)	23
Sugars (g)	4
Exchanges	2
Portions	2.5
GI	Low
GL	Low
Protein:carbohydrate ratio	0.33
Fat (g)	29
Saturated fat (g)	6
Unsaturated fat (g)	23
Saturated:unsaturated ratio	0.26
Fibre (g)	9
Sodium (mg)	9
Potassium (mg)	1475
Sodium:potassium ratio	0.01
Gluten free?	Yes

note

Cook extra corn cobs and cut off the kernels to add to salads or fritters.

CHILLI CHICKEN *and* CORIANDER QUESADILLAS

Quesadillas were originally made in Mexico using corn tortillas. This recipe uses barley wraps, which are a source of fibre, naturally low in fat and sodium, and moderate in carbohydrate.

Ingredients

4 x 45 g (1½ oz) wholegrain barley wraps

olive oil spray

150 g (5½ oz) poached skinless chicken breast fillet, shredded

2 tablespoons bottled jalapeños, drained and chopped

½ red onion, thinly sliced

1 handful coriander (cilantro) leaves, chopped, plus extra to serve

30 g (1 oz/⅓ cup) grated reduced-fat cheddar cheese

60 g (2¼ oz/2 cups) watercress sprigs

125 g (4½ oz) baby roma (plum) tomatoes, halved

2 teaspoons white balsamic vinegar

lemon wedges, to serve

Method

1 Spray one side of two of the wraps with olive oil and place on a board, oiled side down. Divide the chicken, jalapeños, onion, coriander and cheese between the wraps. Top with the remaining wraps and spray them with oil.

2 Heat a non-stick frying pan over medium heat. Carefully place one quesadilla in the pan and cook for 2–3 minutes on each side or until the outside is golden and the cheese has melted. Slide the quesadilla onto a plate and keep warm while you cook the other quesadilla.

3 Combine the watercress and tomato halves in a small bowl, then drizzle with the vinegar. Cut the quesadillas into wedges and serve with the extra coriander, lemon wedges and salad.

Serves 4
Preparation 10 minutes
Cooking 15 minutes

Nutrition	Per serve
Energy (kJ)	920
Protein (g)	18
Carbohydrate (g)	12.5
Starches (g)	11
Sugars (g)	1.5
Exchanges	1
Portions	1
GI	Low
GL	Low
Protein:carbohydrate ratio	1.44
Fat (g)	8
Saturated fat (g)	2.5
Unsaturated fat (g)	5.5
Saturated:unsaturated ratio	0.46
Fibre (g)	3
Sodium (mg)	200
Potassium (mg)	375
Sodium:potassium ratio	0.53
Gluten free?	No

CHICKEN *and* QUINOA PATTIES

Minced chicken can be drier than other minced meats, so quinoa is added to these patties to provide some moisture. Coating the patties with quinoa gives a crunchy texture, while the insides remain tender.

Ingredients

150 g (5½ oz/¾ cup) tri-coloured quinoa, rinsed

140 g (5 oz/1 cup) frozen peas, thawed

400 g (14 oz) lean minced (ground) chicken

2 spring onions (scallions), thinly sliced

1 tablespoon chopped tarragon leaves, plus extra to serve

½ teaspoon celery seeds

¼ teaspoon ground white pepper

olive oil spray

200 g (7 oz) mixed salad leaves

1 small Lebanese (short) cucumber, sliced

250 g (9 oz) cherry tomatoes, halved

lemon wedges, to serve

reduced-fat plain yoghurt, to serve (optional)

Method

1 Combine the quinoa and 375 ml (13 fl oz/1½ cups) water in a small saucepan over high heat. Bring to the boil, then reduce the heat, cover and simmer for 15 minutes or until the quinoa is tender and the water has been absorbed. Spread the quinoa over a baking tray to cool for 15 minutes.

2 Put the peas and 500 ml (17 fl oz/2 cups) water in a small saucepan. Bring to the boil over high heat and cook for 3–4 minutes or until the peas are soft. Drain and roughly mash with the back of a fork.

3 Put half the quinoa in a bowl and add the peas, chicken, spring onions, tarragon, celery seeds and white pepper. Mix until combined, then divide the mixture into 12 portions and use your hands to roll and shape them into patties. Press the patties into the remaining quinoa to coat. Put the patties on a baking tray, cover and refrigerate for 30 minutes.

4 Spray a large non-stick frying pan with olive oil and place over medium–low heat. Cook the patties in batches for 3–4 minutes on each side or until golden and cooked through.

5 Serve the patties with the salad leaves, cucumber, tomatoes and extra tarragon leaves, with the lemon wedges and yoghurt (if using) on the side.

Serves 4
Preparation 20 minutes +
15 minutes cooling and
30 minutes chilling
Cooking 35 minutes

Nutrition	Per serve
Energy (kJ)	1440
Protein (g)	28
Carbohydrate (g)	30
Starches (g)	26
Sugars (g)	4
Exchanges	2
Portions	3
GI	Low
GL	Low
Protein:carbohydrate ratio	0.93
Fat (g)	11
Saturated fat (g)	3
Unsaturated fat (g)	8
Saturated:unsaturated ratio	0.38
Fibre (g)	7
Sodium (mg)	100
Potassium (mg)	890
Sodium:potassium ratio	0.11
Gluten free?	Yes

notes

You can freeze the uncooked patties for up to 3 months, wrapped in plastic wrap or placed in resealable plastic bags. Try other combinations such as lamb and mint or pork and sage.

SPICED PORK *and* WATER CHESTNUT DUMPLING SOUP

Packed with low-GI carbohydrates and dietary fibre, this soup is also high in potassium. Minced chicken can be used instead of the pork, and you can add a little more chilli for a spicier soup.

Ingredients

400 g (14 oz) lean minced (ground) pork

230 g (8 oz) tinned water chestnuts, drained and finely chopped

2 spring onions (scallions), finely chopped, plus extra slices to serve

2 garlic cloves, crushed

1 long red chilli, seeded and finely chopped

250 ml (9 fl oz/1 cup) salt-reduced chicken stock

1 star anise

¼ teaspoon ground white pepper

1 tablespoon salt-reduced soy sauce

30 g (1 oz) piece fresh ginger, cut into matchsticks

125 g (4½ oz) baby corn, halved lengthways

150 g (5½ oz) Chinese cabbage (wong bok), shredded

400 g (14 oz) choy sum, cut into short lengths

200 g (7 oz) dried egg noodles

1 small handful coriander (cilantro) leaves, to serve

Method

1 Put the pork, water chestnuts, chopped spring onions, garlic and red chilli in a bowl and mix until combined. Season the mixture with freshly ground black pepper. Roll into 24 balls, using 1 tablespoon of the mixture for each.

2 Combine the stock, star anise, white pepper and 1 litre (35 fl oz/4 cups) water in a large saucepan. Bring to the boil over medium–high heat. Add the dumplings, reduce the heat to low and simmer for 8–10 minutes or until the dumplings are cooked through. Stir in the soy sauce, ginger, baby corn, Chinese cabbage and choy sum, and simmer for a further 2 minutes.

3 Add the noodles to a saucepan of boiling water. Cook for 3 minutes, stirring with a fork to separate the noodles, then drain.

4 Divide the noodles among four bowls. Ladle the soup and dumplings onto the noodles and serve sprinkled with the coriander leaves and spring onion slices.

Serves 4
Preparation 20 minutes
Cooking 20 minutes

Nutrition	Per serve
Energy (kJ)	1840
Protein (g)	34
Carbohydrate (g)	61
Starches (g)	56
Sugars (g)	5
Exchanges	4
Portions	6
GI	Low
GL	High
Protein:carbohydrate ratio	0.56
Fat (g)	3.5
Saturated fat (g)	1
Unsaturated fat (g)	2.5
Saturated:unsaturated ratio	0.4
Fibre (g)	13.5
Sodium (mg)	425
Potassium (mg)	1420
Sodium:potassium ratio	0.3
Gluten free?	No

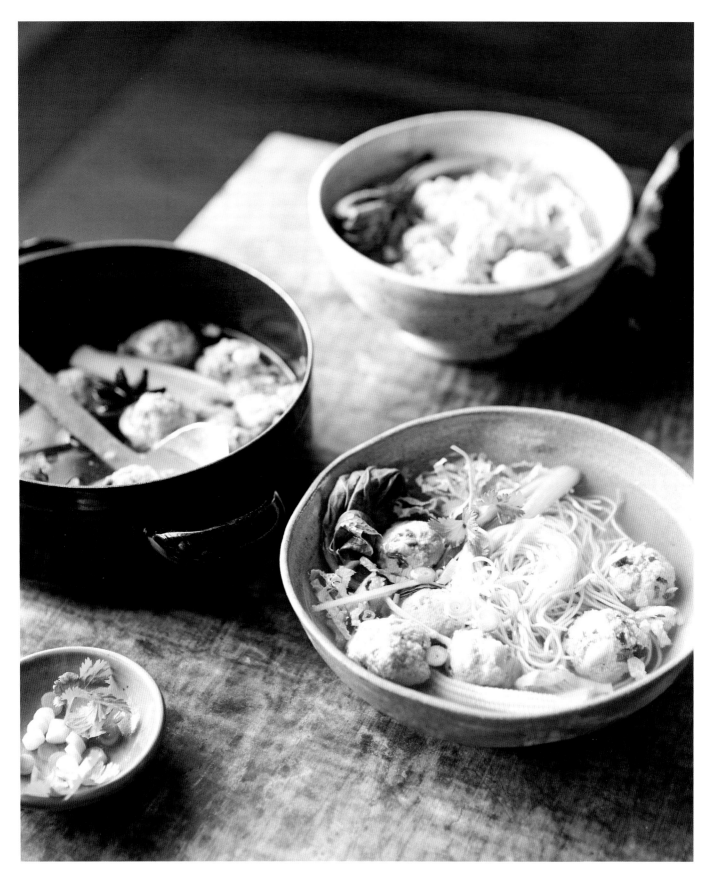

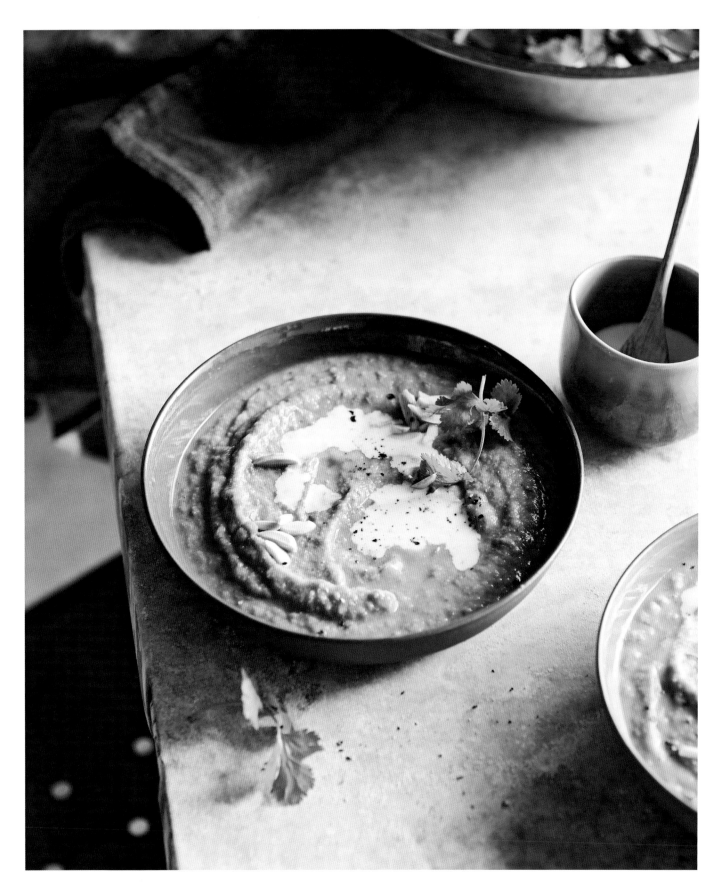

SPICED CAULIFLOWER *and* LENTIL SOUP

This vegetarian soup is moderate in carbohydrate, low in salt and high
in dietary fibre and potassium. Make a double batch of the soup and
freeze half for another meal.

Ingredients

olive oil spray
1 leek, pale part only, chopped
2 garlic cloves, chopped
1 long green chilli, chopped
2 teaspoons ground coriander
2 teaspoons ground cumin
¼ teaspoon ground turmeric
350 g (12 oz) cauliflower
    florets
110 g (3¾ oz/½ cup) green
    lentils, rinsed
1 tablespoon reduced-fat
    coconut milk
1 tablespoon toasted slivered
    almonds
1 small handful coriander
    (cilantro) leaves

Method

1 Spray a large saucepan with olive oil and place
over medium heat. Add the leek and cook, stirring,
for 2 minutes or until softened. Add the garlic, chilli,
ground coriander, cumin and turmeric, and stir for
1 minute or until aromatic.

2 Add the cauliflower florets, green lentils and 1 litre
(35 fl oz/4 cups) water. Cover the pan and cook for
30–35 minutes or until the cauliflower and lentils
are tender.

3 Using a stick blender, blend the soup until smooth.

4 Ladle the soup into bowls and serve topped with
the coconut milk, almonds, coriander leaves and
freshly ground black pepper.

Serves 2
Preparation 10 minutes
Cooking 40 minutes

Nutrition	Per serve
Energy (kJ)	1295
Protein (g)	22
Carbohydrate (g)	32
Starches (g)	22
Sugars (g)	10
Exchanges	2
Portions	3
GI	Low
GL	Low
Protein:carbohydrate ratio	0.69
Fat (g)	7
Saturated fat (g)	0.5
Unsaturated fat (g)	6.5
Saturated:unsaturated ratio	0.08
Fibre (g)	16
Sodium (mg)	70
Potassium (mg)	1350
Sodium:potassium ratio	0.05
Gluten free?	Yes

notes

*Try using Moroccan spice powder and 1 tablespoon of harissa paste instead of the
ground cumin and coriander. Substitute the lentils with diced orange sweet potato.*

CHICKEN POACHED *in* FRAGRANT ASIAN BROTH

This flavoursome broth creates a tasty soup base. For maximum nutritional benefit, make the broth a day ahead, refrigerate it overnight and then scoop off any solidified fat from the surface before reheating.

Ingredients

2 x 200 g (7 oz) skinless chicken breast fillets
50 g (1¾ oz) piece fresh ginger, sliced, plus 40 g (1½ oz) shredded ginger to serve
50 g (1¾ oz) galangal, sliced
4 spring onions (scallions), sliced, plus extra slices to serve
4 kaffir lime leaves, torn
1 lemongrass stem, bruised
1 star anise
1 long red chilli, halved
½ cinnamon stick
2 garlic cloves
100 g (3½ oz) rice stick noodles
115 g (4 oz) baby corn, halved lengthways
200 g (7 oz) snake (yard-long) beans, trimmed
100 g (3½ oz) snow peas (mangetout), thinly sliced
Vietnamese mint leaves, to serve
lime cheeks, to serve

Method

1 Pour 1 litre (35 fl oz/4 cups) water into a large saucepan and add the chicken, sliced ginger, galangal, spring onions, lime leaves, lemongrass, star anise, chilli, cinnamon and garlic. Place over low heat, cover and simmer for 15–20 minutes or until the chicken is cooked through.

2 Meanwhile, put the noodles in a heatproof bowl and cover with boiling water. Leave to soak for 5 minutes or until softened, then drain.

3 Use a slotted spoon to lift the chicken from the broth. Strain the broth and return it to the pan. Thickly slice the chicken.

4 Add the baby corn and snake beans to the broth and cook for 2 minutes, then add the snow peas. Cook for a further 1 minute or until the vegetables are tender.

5 Divide the noodles, chicken, corn, beans and snow peas among four bowls and ladle over the broth. Top with the mint leaves and extra ginger and spring onions, and serve with lime cheeks.

Serves 4
Preparation 15 minutes
Cooking 25 minutes

Nutrition	Per serve
Energy (kJ)	1245
Protein (g)	27
Carbohydrate (g)	31
Starches (g)	28
Sugars (g)	3
Exchanges	2
Portions	3
GI	Low
GL	Low
Protein:carbohydrate ratio	0.87
Fat (g)	6
Saturated fat (g)	2
Unsaturated fat (g)	4
Saturated:unsaturated ratio	0.5
Fibre (g)	6
Sodium (mg)	160
Potassium (mg)	750
Sodium:potassium ratio	0.21
Gluten free?	Yes

notes

Make double the quantity of the poaching broth, then freeze the cooled broth to use as a flavoursome stock. For added heat, substitute the long red chilli with a hotter variety such as small bird's eye chillies — the smaller the chilli, the hotter it will be.

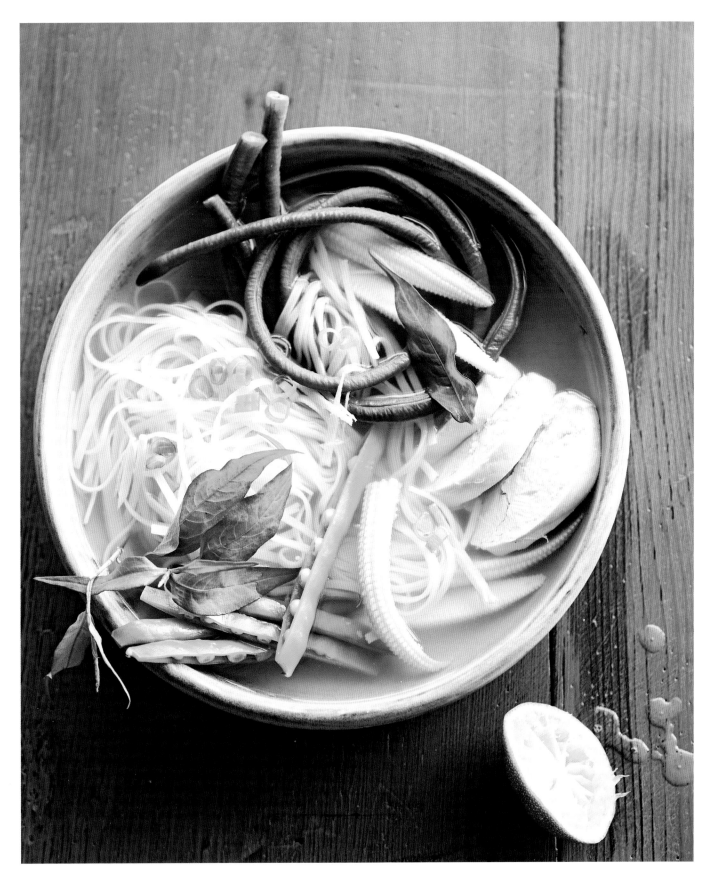

MINESTRONE *with* BARLEY *and* CROUTONS

Barley contains soluble fibre, which helps slow the absorption of glucose.
This ancient grain has a low GI, is naturally low in fat and is filled with
antioxidants and vitamins.

Ingredients

195 g (6¾ oz/1 cup) dried
   cannellini beans, soaked
   overnight
1 tablespoon olive oil
2 brown onions, finely
   chopped
2 celery stalks, thinly sliced
2 carrots, finely chopped
1 kg (2 lb 4 oz) ripe tomatoes,
   diced
2 garlic cloves, crushed
250 ml (9 fl oz/1 cup) salt-
   reduced vegetable stock
12 x 5 g (⅛ oz) slices wholemeal
   (whole-wheat) baguette
olive oil spray
100 g (3½ oz/½ cup) barley
1 small handful basil leaves,
   shredded

Method

1 Drain and rinse the soaked cannellini beans.

2 Heat the olive oil in a large saucepan over
medium heat. Cook the onions, celery and carrots,
stirring, for 5 minutes or until softened. Add the
tomatoes and garlic, and stir for 2 minutes or until
softened. Add the soaked cannellini beans, stock
and 1.25 litres (44 fl oz/5 cups) water. Cover, reduce
the heat to low and simmer for 20 minutes.

3 Meanwhile, preheat the grill (broiler) to high. Put
the baguette slices on a baking tray and lightly spray
with olive oil. Cook for 2–3 minutes on each side or
until golden.

4 Stir the barley into the soup and cook for a further
20 minutes.

5 Ladle the soup into bowls and serve topped with
the croutons and basil.

Serves 4
Preparation 20 minutes +
overnight soaking
Cooking 50 minutes

Nutrition	Per serve
Energy (kJ)	1195
Protein (g)	12
Carbohydrate (g)	38
Starches (g)	28
Sugars (g)	10
Exchanges	2.5
Portions	4
GI	Low
GL	Medium
Protein:carbohydrate ratio	0.31
Fat (g)	7
Saturated fat (g)	1
Unsaturated fat (g)	6
Saturated:unsaturated ratio	0.17
Fibre (g)	12
Sodium (mg)	290
Potassium (mg)	1025
Sodium:potassium ratio	0.28
Gluten free?	No

SATAY PORK SKEWERS *with* WILD RICE SALAD

Wild rice is actually not a type of rice, but an aquatic grain. Low in fat and a source of dietary fibre, it is gluten free, and has a chewy, nutty texture that works well in salads.

Ingredients

400 g (14 oz) piece pork fillet
1 tablespoon unsalted peanuts
1 teaspoon coriander seeds
1 teaspoon cumin seeds
2 tablespoons lime juice
20 g (¾ oz) palm sugar, grated
½ teaspoon ground turmeric
½ teaspoon garam masala
1 garlic clove, crushed
olive oil spray
1 spring onion (scallion),
    thinly sliced
lime wedges, to serve

Wild rice salad

100 g (3½ oz) wild rice
2 Lebanese (short) cucumbers,
    peeled into ribbons
5 radishes, thinly sliced
2 spring onions (scallions),
    thinly sliced
2 tablespoons white balsamic
    vinegar
1 tablespoon avocado oil
1 tablespoon unsalted peanuts,
    chopped
2 tablespoons chopped dill

Method

1 Slice the pork fillet into long, thin strips and put in a bowl. Grind the peanuts with the coriander seeds and cumin seeds in a spice mill or use a mortar and pestle. Add the peanut mixture to the pork along with the lime juice, palm sugar, turmeric, garam masala and garlic, and stir well. Cover and refrigerate for 2 hours.

2 To make the wild rice salad, put the rice in a saucepan with enough water to cover it. Bring to the boil, then reduce the heat to low and simmer for 40–45 minutes or until the rice is tender and just starting to curl. Drain and transfer to a bowl.

3 Mix the cucumbers, radishes and spring onions through the rice. Whisk the vinegar and avocado oil in a small bowl, pour over the salad and mix well. Set the salad aside for 15 minutes for the rice to soak up the dressing.

4 Preheat a chargrill pan or barbecue to high. Thread the pork onto eight skewers, spray with olive oil and cook for 2 minutes on each side or until golden and cooked through.

5 Sprinkle the chopped peanuts and dill over the salad and serve with the pork skewers, spring onion and lime wedges.

Serves 4

Preparation 20 minutes +
2 hours marinating
Cooking 50 minutes

Nutrition	Per serve
Energy (kJ)	1325
Protein (g)	28
Carbohydrate (g)	25
Starches (g)	17
Sugars (g)	8
Exchanges	1.5
Portions	2.5
GI	Low
GL	Low
Protein:carbohydrate ratio	1.12
Fat (g)	10
Saturated fat (g)	1
Unsaturated fat (g)	9
Saturated:unsaturated ratio	0.11
Fibre (g)	4
Sodium (mg)	70
Potassium (mg)	660
Sodium:potassium ratio	0.11
Gluten free?	Yes

notes

If you are using wooden skewers, soak them in water for 30 minutes before use to prevent them from burning during cooking. Chicken can be used instead of pork if preferred.

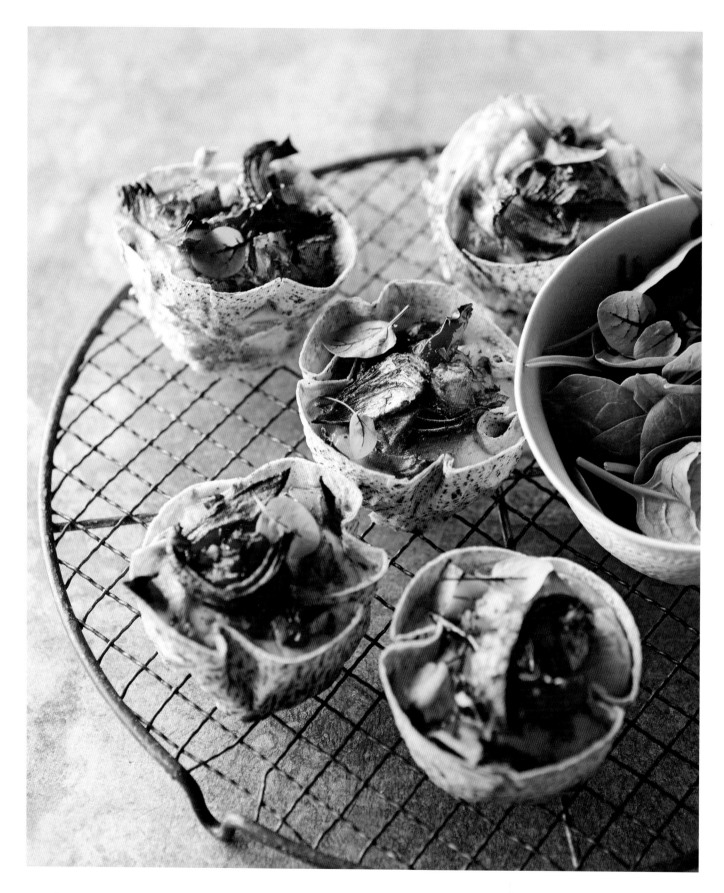

SPANISH TORTILLA PIES

To save time, make these tortilla pies a day ahead. Take any left-over pies for lunch the next day with a mixed salad.

Ingredients

1 large red capsicum (pepper), thickly sliced

1 large lower-GI potato, such as Carisma, diced

1 large red onion, cut into thin wedges

olive oil spray

2 teaspoons smoked Spanish paprika

6 x 30 g (1 oz) low-sodium sorj rye wraps

4 eggs, plus 2 eggwhites

125 ml (4 fl oz/½ cup) skim milk

2 tablespoons parsley leaves, finely chopped

250 g (9 oz) mixed salad leaves

2 teaspoons white balsamic vinegar

Method

1 Preheat the oven to 180°C (350°F). Line a baking tray with baking paper. Spread the capsicum, potato and onion over the tray, spray with olive oil and sprinkle with the paprika. Bake for 30 minutes or until the vegetables have softened.

2 Using a 14 cm (5½ inch) round cutter, cut a circle from each wrap. Lightly spray one side of the circles with olive oil and gently press the oiled side into six 185 ml (6 fl oz/¾ cup) capacity muffin holes.

3 Divide the roasted vegetables among the muffin holes. Whisk the eggs, eggwhites and milk together in a small bowl. Pour over the vegetables, sprinkle with the parsley and bake for 25 minutes or until the pies are golden and set.

4 Drizzle the salad leaves with the white balsamic vinegar and serve with the hot pies.

Serves 6
Preparation 20 minutes
Cooking 55 minutes

Nutrition	Per serve
Energy (kJ)	930
Protein (g)	14
Carbohydrate (g)	28
Starches (g)	23
Sugars (g)	5
Exchanges	2
Portions	3
GI	Medium
GL	Medium
Protein:carbohydrate ratio	0.5
Fat (g)	5
Saturated fat (g)	1.5
Unsaturated fat (g)	3.5
Saturated:unsaturated ratio	0.43
Fibre (g)	4
Sodium (mg)	235
Potassium (mg)	570
Sodium:potassium ratio	0.41
Gluten free?	No

notes

Gently heat the wraps in the microwave before cutting them into rounds — this will make it easy to shape them into the muffin holes. Sprinkle each tortilla with a small quantity of Spanish manchego cheese before baking. Manchego is a sheep's cheese with a delicate nutty flavour.

CHICKEN *and* SPINACH KATAIFI PASTRY PARCELS

A little of this fine pastry goes a long way. Freeze any left-over pastry in
a resealable plastic bag. Try using other fillings in the pastry such as lean
turkey breast, ricotta cheese and a few dried cranberries.

Ingredients

300 g (10½ oz) skinless
chicken breast fillets

250 g (9 oz) packet frozen
spinach, thawed

2 spring onions (scallions),
finely chopped

2 tablespoons low-fat
cottage cheese

2 tablespoons extra light
sour cream

1 garlic clove, crushed

1 tablespoon pine nuts,
toasted

½ teaspoon finely grated
lemon zest

pinch of freshly grated
nutmeg

60 g (2¼ oz) kataifi pastry

olive oil spray

200 g (7 oz) mixed salad
leaves

lemon wedges, to serve

Method

1 Preheat the oven to 200°C (400°F). Line a baking
tray with baking paper.

2 Slice the chicken lengthways into 16 strips about
3 x 10 cm (1¼ x 4 inches) and 5 mm (¼ inch) thick.
Lay the strips flat on a clean work surface.

3 Squeeze the liquid from the spinach and put the
spinach in a bowl with the spring onions, cottage
cheese, sour cream, garlic, pine nuts, lemon zest
and nutmeg.

4 Put a spoonful of the spinach mixture on each
chicken strip and roll up to form a log. Wrap a small
amount of pastry around each roll and arrange on
the prepared tray. Spray with olive oil and bake for
15 minutes or until the pastry is golden and the
chicken is cooked through.

5 Serve the pastry parcels with the mixed salad
leaves and lemon wedges.

Serves 4

Preparation 25 minutes
Cooking 15 minutes

Nutrition	Per serve
Energy (kJ)	975
Protein (g)	23
Carbohydrate (g)	10
Starches (g)	8
Sugars (g)	2
Exchanges	0.5
Portions	1
GI	Low
GL	Low
Protein:carbohydrate ratio	2.3
Fat (g)	9.5
Saturated fat (g)	2.5
Unsaturated fat (g)	7
Saturated:unsaturated ratio	0.36
Fibre (g)	6
Sodium (mg)	250
Potassium (mg)	570
Sodium:potassium ratio	0.4
Gluten free?	No

note

*Kataifi pastry is a finely shredded pastry that looks like vermicelli. It can be found
in Middle Eastern grocery stores and gourmet delicatessens. If it's unavailable, you
can substitute it with thinly sliced filo pastry.*

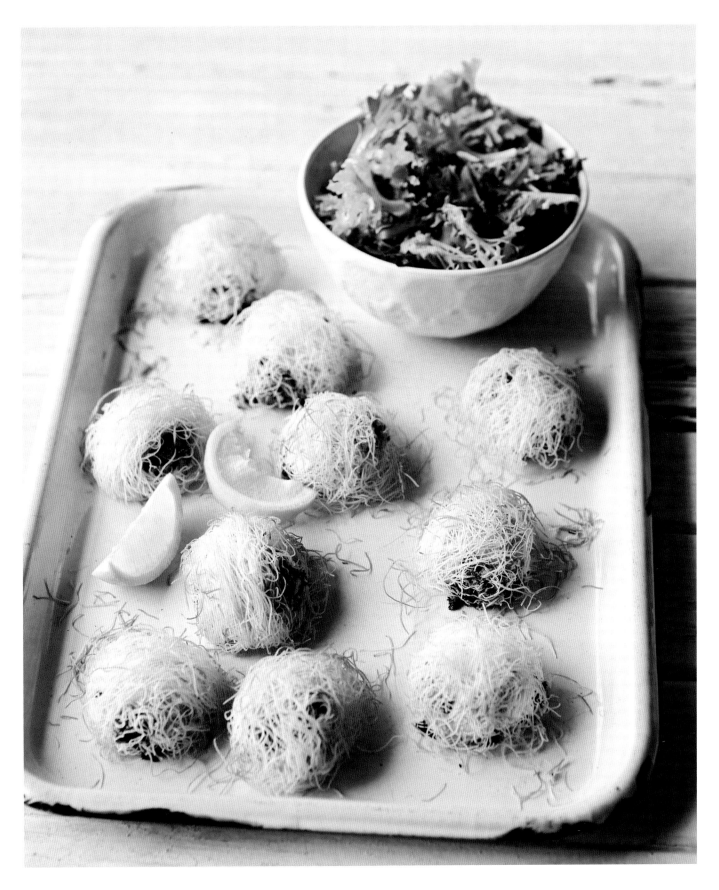

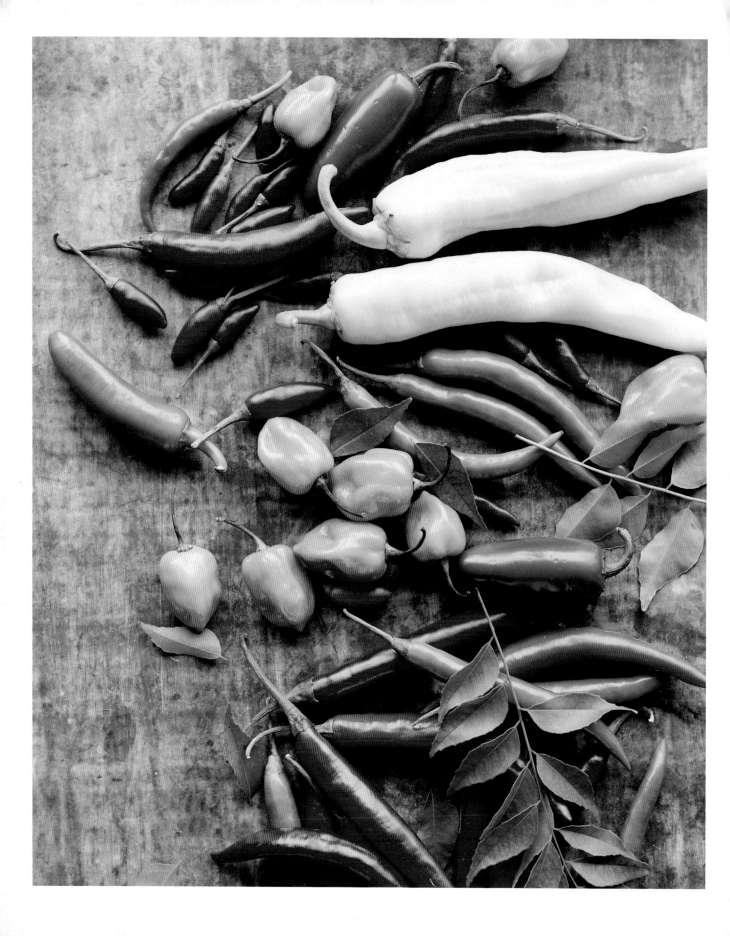

Chapter Three
MEALS FOR TWO

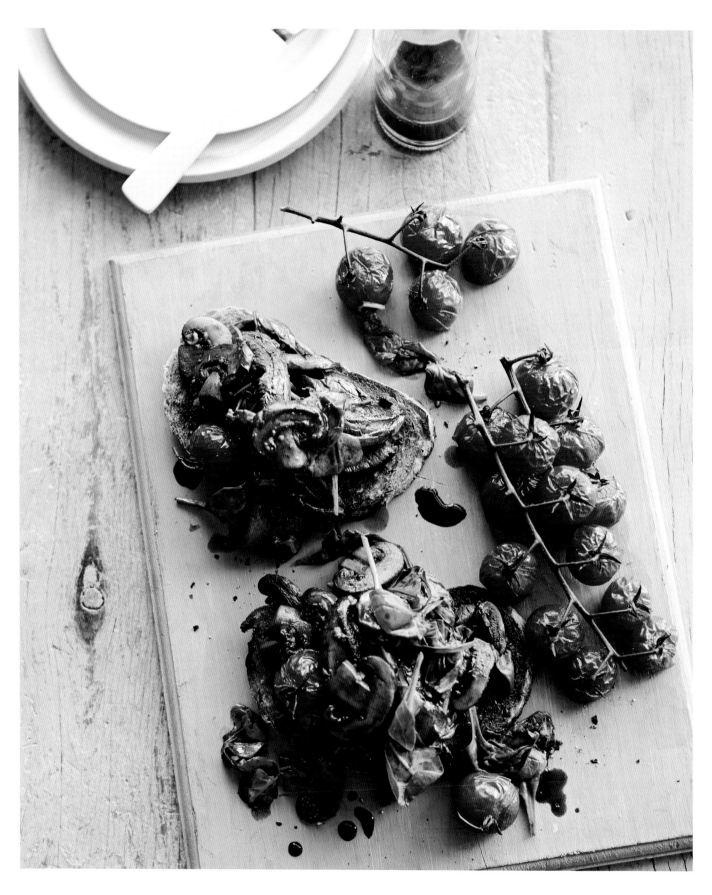

GARLIC MUSHROOMS *and* SPINACH *with* ROASTED TOMATOES

Include other varieties of mushrooms or add a poached egg to turn this into a satisfying brunch meal that's high in fibre, potassium and flavour.

Ingredients

250 g (9 oz) cherry tomatoes on the vine
olive oil spray
250 g (9 oz) Swiss brown mushrooms, sliced
150 g (5½ oz) flat mushrooms, sliced
2 garlic cloves, crushed
80 g (2¾ oz/1¾ cups) baby English spinach leaves
1 tablespoon balsamic vinegar
2 x 30 g (1 oz) slices wholegrain sourdough toast

Method

1 Preheat the oven to 200°C (400°F). Put the tomatoes on a baking tray and spray with olive oil. Bake for 10 minutes or until the tomatoes are just starting to collapse.

2 While the tomatoes are cooking, spray a large non-stick frying pan with olive oil and place over medium heat. Cook the mushrooms, stirring, for 5 minutes or until tender. Add the garlic and cook for 1 minute or until fragrant. Add the spinach and pour in the balsamic vinegar. Cook for 2 minutes or until the spinach has wilted.

3 Spoon the mushrooms and spinach onto the sourdough toast and sprinkle with freshly ground black pepper. Serve with the tomatoes on the side.

Serves 2
Preparation 10 minutes
Cooking 10 minutes

Nutrition	Per serve
Energy (kJ)	790
Protein (g)	12
Carbohydrate (g)	22
Starches (g)	5
Sugars (g)	17
Exchanges	1.5
Portions	2
GI	Low
GL	Low
Protein:carbohydrate ratio	0.55
Fat (g)	3
Saturated fat (g)	0.3
Unsaturated fat (g)	2.7
Saturated:unsaturated ratio	0.11
Fibre (g)	10
Sodium (mg)	230
Potassium (mg)	1210
Sodium:potassium ratio	0.19
Gluten free?	No

PORK, PINEAPPLE *and* MINT RICE SALAD

Double the quantities and serve the salad on a platter for entertaining, or use the leftovers for lunch the next day. You can spice up the salad by sprinkling some chopped chillies over the top.

Ingredients

100 g (3½ oz/½ cup) Doongara low-GI brown rice

olive oil spray

200 g (7 oz) lean minced (ground) pork

1 small red capsicum (pepper), thinly sliced

150 g (5½ oz/2 cups) shredded cabbage

2 spring onions (scallions), sliced

30 g (1 oz) piece fresh ginger, grated

60 g (2¼ oz) mixed salad leaves

100 g (3½ oz) chopped pineapple

1 small handful mint leaves

2 small handfuls coriander (cilantro) leaves

½ Lebanese (short) cucumber, sliced into matchsticks

60 g (2¼ oz) snow peas (mangetout), thinly sliced

60 ml (2 fl oz/¼ cup) lime juice

Method

1 Rinse the rice under cold water, then transfer to a small saucepan with 250 ml (9 fl oz/1 cup) water. Bring to the boil over high heat, then reduce the heat to low, cover and cook for 15–20 minutes or until the rice is tender. Remove from the heat and stand for 5 minutes. Fluff with a fork before using.

2 Meanwhile, lightly spray a large non-stick frying pan with olive oil and place over medium–high heat. Cook the pork, stirring and breaking up any lumps, for 8–10 minutes or until browned. Add the capsicum, cabbage, spring onions and ginger, and stir for 1 minute or until the vegetables start to wilt.

3 Divide the rice between two serving bowls. Spoon the pork and vegetable mixture over the rice. Top with the salad leaves, pineapple, mint, coriander, cucumber and snow peas. Pour the lime juice over the salad and serve.

Serves 2
Preparation 15 minutes
Cooking 20 minutes

Nutrition	Per serve
Energy (kJ)	1710
Protein (g)	30
Carbohydrate (g)	51
Starches (g)	40
Sugars (g)	11
Exchanges	3.5
Portions	5
GI	Low
GL	Low
Protein:carbohydrate ratio	0.59
Fat (g)	7
Saturated fat (g)	2
Unsaturated fat (g)	5
Saturated:unsaturated ratio	0.4
Fibre (g)	9
Sodium (mg)	100
Potassium (mg)	1385
Sodium:potassium ratio	0.07
Gluten free?	Yes

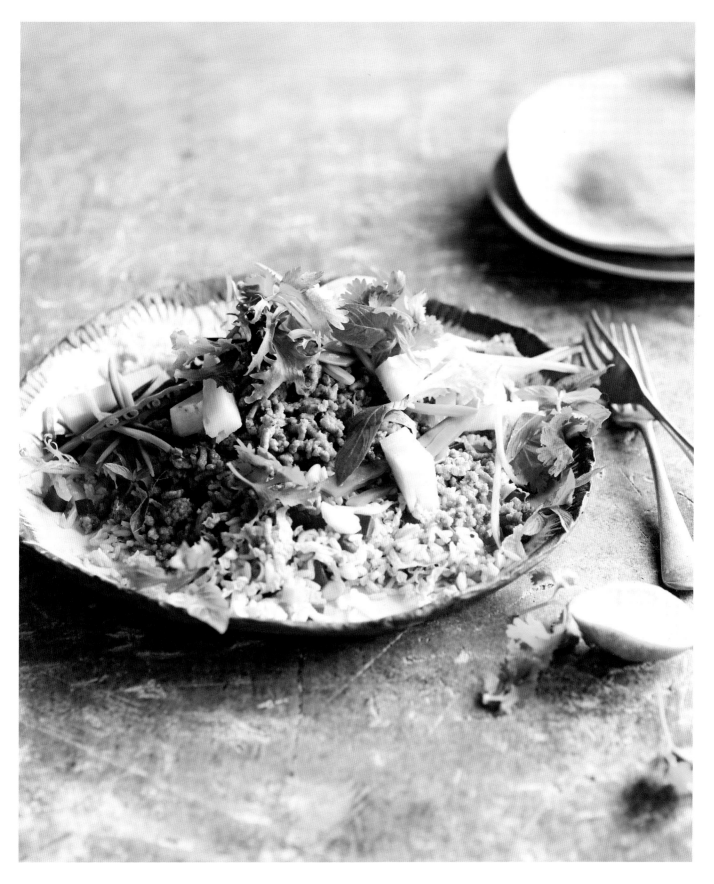

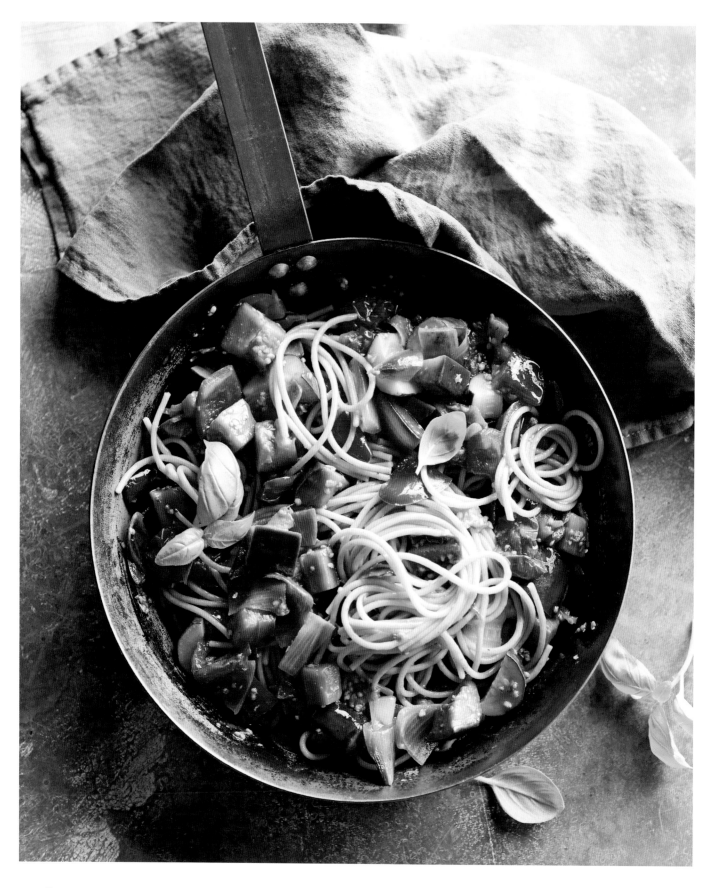

SPELT SPAGHETTI *with* RATATOUILLE

This colourful dish is high in low-GI carbohydrate and dietary fibre to keep you feeling fuller for longer. You can also use regular wheat spaghetti. For a gluten-free option, use rice pasta or another gluten-free pasta.

Ingredients

olive oil spray
1 red onion, roughly chopped
1 eggplant (aubergine), chopped
1 red capsicum (pepper), chopped
2 large zucchini (courgettes), chopped
2 garlic cloves, crushed
250 g (9 oz) cherry tomatoes, halved
140 g (5 oz) spelt spaghetti
1 small handful basil leaves, to serve

Method

1 Spray a large non-stick frying pan with olive oil and place over medium–high heat. Cook the onion, stirring, for 2 minutes or until softened. Stir in the eggplant, capsicum, zucchini and garlic, and cook, stirring occasionally, for 8 minutes.

2 Stir in the tomatoes and 250 ml (9 fl oz/1 cup) water, and cook for a further 2 minutes or until the tomatoes have softened and the other vegetables are tender. Remove the pan from the heat.

3 While the vegetables are cooking, bring a large saucepan of water to the boil and cook the pasta for 8–10 minutes or until al dente.

4 Drain the pasta, add it to the ratatouille and gently toss to combine. Serve the pasta and ratatouille with the basil scattered over the top.

Serves 2
Preparation 15 minutes
Cooking 15 minutes

Nutrition	Per serve
Energy (kJ)	1495
Protein (g)	14
Carbohydrate (g)	62
Starches (g)	49
Sugars (g)	13
Exchanges	4
Portions	6
GI	Low
GL	Low
Protein:carbohydrate ratio	0.23
Fat (g)	3
Saturated fat (g)	0.3
Unsaturated fat (g)	2.7
Saturated:unsaturated ratio	0.11
Fibre (g)	12
Sodium (mg)	30
Potassium (mg)	1085
Sodium:potassium ratio	0.03
Gluten free?	No

TERIYAKI SALMON *with* SOBA NOODLES *and* PICKLED VEGETABLES

Pickling vegetables can improve the overall flavour and make the vegetables easier to digest, boosting the gut's good bacteria. The pickled vegetables can be made up to 3 days ahead and stored in an airtight container in the fridge.

Ingredients

2 tablespoons sake
1 tablespoon salt-reduced soy sauce
1 tablespoon rice vinegar
1 tablespoon mirin
2 teaspoons Splenda sweetener
2 x 150 g (5½ oz) skinless salmon fillets
100 g (3½ oz) no-added-salt dried soba noodles
2 tablespoons cold green tea
½ teaspoon sesame oil
2 spring onions (scallions), thinly sliced
1 teaspoon sesame seeds, toasted
250 g (9 oz) snow peas (mangetout), steamed

Pickled vegetables

60 ml (2 fl oz/¼ cup) rice vinegar
1 teaspoon Splenda sweetener
1 carrot, cut into matchsticks
½ daikon (white radish), cut into matchsticks
1 Lebanese (short) cucumber, cut into matchsticks

Method

1 Combine the sake, soy sauce, vinegar, mirin and sweetener in a small saucepan over low heat. Cook, stirring, for 1–2 minutes or until the sweetener has dissolved. Set aside to cool for 10 minutes.

2 Put the salmon in a glass bowl and pour over the marinade, reserving 1 tablespoon. Cover and marinate in the refrigerator for 30 minutes.

3 To make the pickled vegetables, pour the vinegar and sweetener into a glass bowl. Stir for 1 minute or until the sweetener has dissolved, then add the carrot, daikon and cucumber, and toss to combine. Cover and refrigerate for 30 minutes.

4 Cook the noodles in a saucepan of boiling water for 4 minutes or according to the packet directions. Drain and rinse under cold water. Transfer to a bowl. Stir the reserved marinade, green tea and sesame oil into the noodles. Set aside until needed.

5 Heat a non-stick frying pan over medium heat. Remove the salmon from the marinade, reserving the marinade. Cook for 3 minutes on each side, adding the reserved marinade for the last minute of cooking.

6 Divide the noodles between two bowls and top with the salmon, spring onions and sesame seeds. Serve with the pickled vegetables and snow peas.

Serves 2

Preparation 30 minutes +
10 minutes cooling and
30 minutes marinating
Cooking 15 minutes

Nutrition	Per serve
Energy (kJ)	2115
Protein (g)	39
Carbohydrate (g)	24
Starches (g)	15
Sugars (g)	9
Exchanges	1.5
Portions	2.5
GI	Low
GL	Low
Protein:carbohydrate ratio	1.6
Fat (g)	23
Saturated fat (g)	6
Unsaturated fat (g)	17
Saturated:unsaturated ratio	0.35
Fibre (g)	6
Sodium (mg)	470
Potassium (mg)	1220
Sodium:potassium ratio	0.39
Gluten free?	Yes

notes

Sake is a Japanese rice wine that can be purchased from most liquor stores. Mirin and rice vinegar can be found in large supermarkets or in Asian grocery stores. You can substitute chicken for the salmon if preferred.

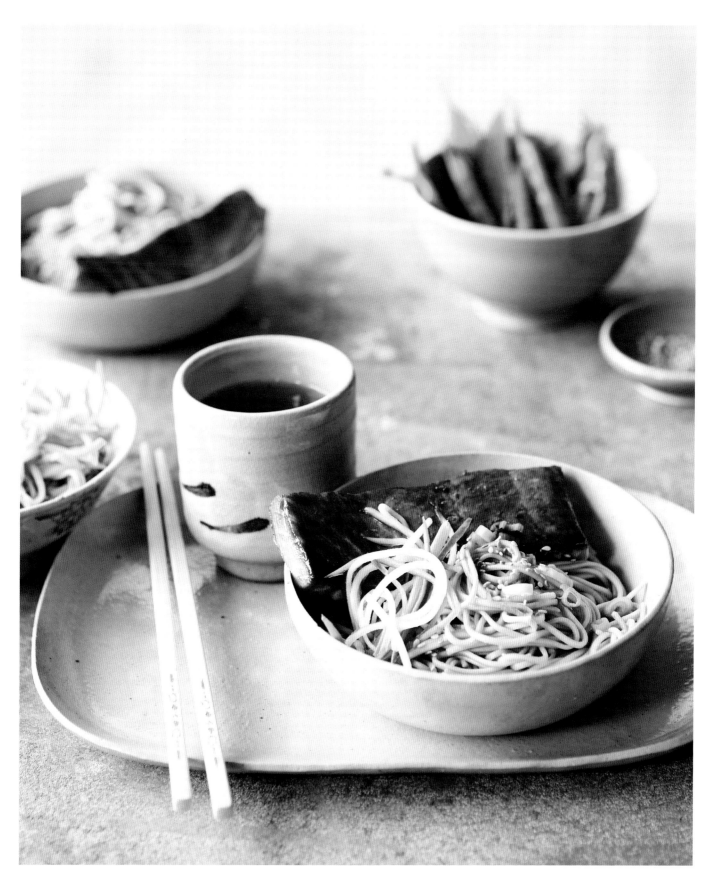

Meals for Two 127

CHIMICHURRI CHICKEN
with TOMATO SALAD

Chimichurri is a tangy sauce made from chopped mixed herbs and spices, traditionally served with barbecued meats. This lower-carbohydrate option is an excellent source of dietary fibre and potassium.

Ingredients
250 g (9 oz) chicken
    tenderloins
2 large ripe tomatoes, sliced
1 small red onion, sliced
100 g (3½ oz) mixed salad
    leaves
lemon wedges, to serve

Chimichurri sauce
1 large handful parsley leaves,
    finely chopped
1 small handful coriander
    (cilantro) leaves, finely
    chopped
1 small handful oregano
    leaves, finely chopped
2 garlic cloves, finely chopped
½ teaspoon ground cumin
½ teaspoon chilli powder
2 tablespoons macadamia oil
2 tablespoons white wine
    vinegar

Method
1 To make the chimichurri sauce, mix the parsley, coriander, oregano, garlic, cumin, chilli powder, macadamia oil and white wine vinegar together in a small bowl.

2 Put the chicken tenderloins in a glass bowl. Pour over half the chimichurri sauce and rub the sauce all over the chicken to coat it.

3 Preheat a barbecue or chargrill pan to medium-high. Cook the chicken for 2 minutes on each side or until golden and cooked through. Transfer the chicken to a plate, cover and rest for 5 minutes. Cut the chicken into thick slices.

4 Arrange the tomato and onion slices on two serving plates, top with the chicken and drizzle with the remaining chimichurri sauce. Serve the chicken with the salad leaves and lemon wedges.

Serves 2
Preparation 15 minutes +
5 minutes resting
Cooking 5 minutes

Nutrition	Per serve
Energy (kJ)	1740
Protein (g)	27
Carbohydrate (g)	7
Starches (g)	1
Sugars (g)	6
Exchanges	0.5
Portions	0.5
GI	Low
GL	Low
Protein:carbohydrate ratio	3.9
Fat (g)	28
Saturated fat (g)	6
Unsaturated fat (g)	22
Saturated:unsaturated ratio	0.27
Fibre (g)	8
Sodium (mg)	150
Potassium (mg)	1160
Sodium:potassium ratio	0.13
Gluten free?	Yes

DUKKAH-CRUSTED LAMB CUTLETS
with JEWELLED COUSCOUS

Dukkah is an Egyptian mixture of nuts, seeds and dried spices. It is usually pounded together and used for coating meat or for dipping. Make a double batch and store it in a sealed container in the refrigerator for up to a month.

Ingredients

135 g (4¾ oz/¾ cup) pearl couscous
1 Lebanese (short) cucumber, diced
2 tablespoons goji berries
1 small handful mint leaves
1 small handful parsley leaves
juice and grated zest of 1 lemon
seeds of 1 pomegranate
6 x 50 g (1¾ oz) French-trimmed lamb cutlets
olive oil spray
150 g (5½ oz) low-fat plain yoghurt
lemon wedges, to serve

Dukkah

2 teaspoons coriander seeds
1 teaspoon cumin seeds
1 teaspoon black peppercorns
2 tablespoons hazelnuts, finely chopped
1 teaspoon sesame seeds

Method

1 Put the couscous and 250 ml (9 fl oz/1 cup) water in a saucepan. Bring to the boil, then reduce the heat to low, cover and simmer for 8–10 minutes or until the couscous is tender and the water has been absorbed. Transfer to a large bowl and set aside to cool for 15 minutes.

2 Add the cucumber, goji berries, mint, parsley, lemon juice, lemon zest and pomegranate seeds to the cooled couscous. Toss to combine, cover and refrigerate until required.

3 To make the dukkah, crush the coriander seeds, cumin seeds and peppercorns using a mortar and pestle. Transfer to a small bowl and mix in the hazelnuts and sesame seeds.

4 Spread the dukkah on a plate and press each side of the lamb cutlets into the mixture. Spray a large non-stick frying pan with olive oil and place over medium heat. Cook the cutlets for 2–3 minutes on each side or until browned on the outside and pink on the inside.

5 Serve the cutlets with the couscous, yoghurt and lemon wedges.

Serves 2
Preparation 35 minutes +
15 minutes cooling
Cooking 20 minutes

Nutrition	Per serve
Energy (kJ)	2810
Protein (g)	49
Carbohydrate (g)	68
Starches (g)	52
Sugars (g)	16
Exchanges	4.5
Portions	7
GI	Low
GL	Medium
Protein:carbohydrate ratio	0.72
Fat (g)	19
Saturated fat (g)	6
Unsaturated fat (g)	13
Saturated:unsaturated ratio	0.46
Fibre (g)	8.5
Sodium (mg)	200
Potassium (mg)	1055
Sodium:potassium ratio	0.19
Gluten free?	No

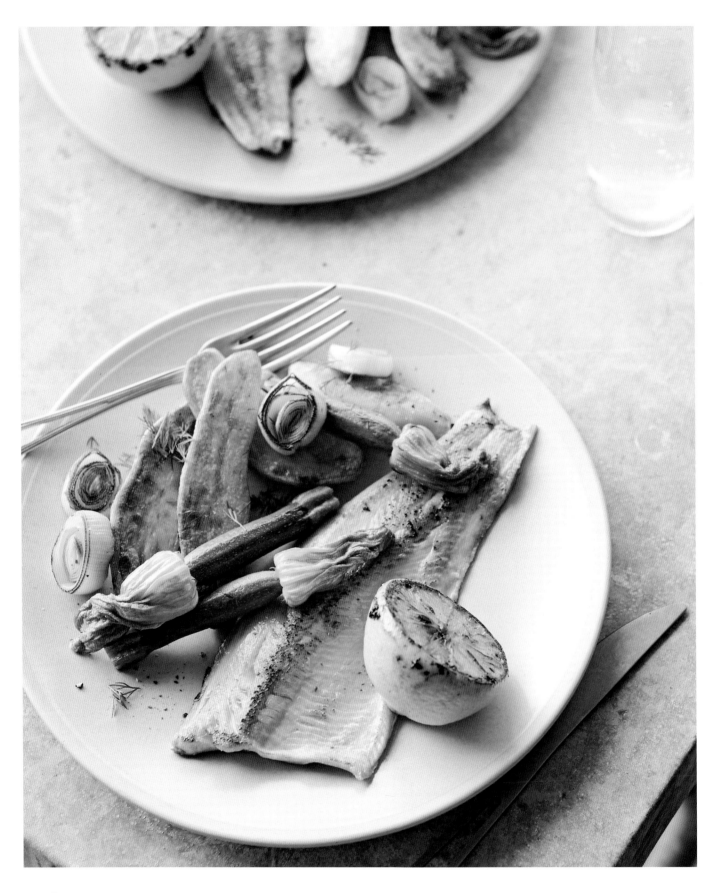

PAN-FRIED RIVER TROUT
with SAUTÉED POTATOES

River trout has a mild flavour that makes it a perfect choice for those who do not like strong fishy flavours. This dish is high in protein, moderate in carbohydrate and a good source of dietary fibre and omega-3 fats.

Ingredients

250 g (9 oz) kipfler (fingerling) potatoes, thickly sliced
olive oil spray
1 leek, pale part only, thickly sliced
1 lemon, halved
2 x 120 g (4¼ oz) freshwater trout fillets
6 zucchini (courgette) flowers
1 small handful dill, chopped

Method

1 Add the potatoes and 750 ml (26 fl oz/3 cups) water to a saucepan. Bring to the boil over high heat, then reduce the heat to medium and cook for 7–8 minutes or until just tender. Drain and set aside until needed.

2 Spray a large non-stick frying pan with olive oil and place over medium–high heat. Cook the leek for 2 minutes. Add the potatoes and cook, stirring, for 3–4 minutes or until golden.

3 Meanwhile, heat another non-stick frying pan over medium–high heat. Put the lemon halves, cut side down, in the pan with the trout and cook for 3–4 minutes or until the trout is golden. Turn and cook for another 3–4 minutes or until the trout is golden and cooked and the lemon is browned and juicy. Add the zucchini flowers for the last 2 minutes of cooking.

4 Serve the trout with the potatoes, leek, zucchini flowers and lemon, sprinkled with the dill and some freshly ground black pepper.

Serves 2
Preparation 10 minutes
Cooking 20 minutes

Nutrition	Per serve
Energy (kJ)	1100
Protein (g)	28
Carbohydrate (g)	20
Starches (g)	16
Sugars (g)	4
Exchanges	1.5
Portions	2
GI	Medium
GL	Low
Protein:carbohydrate ratio	1.4
Fat (g)	6
Saturated fat (g)	1
Unsaturated fat (g)	5
Saturated:unsaturated ratio	0.2
Fibre (g)	6
Sodium (mg)	75
Potassium (mg)	1430
Sodium:potassium ratio	0.05
Gluten free?	Yes

note

If the trout fillets are large, divide one fillet between two people or use the extra fillet for lunch the next day, flaked in a salad.

TURKEY and SAGE BURGERS with ONION and FENNEL RELISH

Proof that it is possible to make healthy, tasty burgers, these are high in protein, moderate in carbohydrate and high in dietary fibre and potassium. Other flavours work well – try chicken and tarragon or pork and coriander.

Ingredients

200 g (7 oz) lean minced (ground) turkey
1 small zucchini (courgette), grated
1 tablespoon sage leaves, finely chopped
¼ teaspoon ground white pepper
¼ teaspoon ground fennel
1 eggwhite
olive oil spray
2 x 60 g (2¼ oz) multigrain bread rolls
20 g (¾ oz) mixed lettuce leaves
1 tomato, sliced
1 Lebanese (short) cucumber, sliced into ribbons

Onion and fennel relish

1 red onion, sliced
1 small fennel bulb, sliced
1 green apple, peeled, cored and chopped
2 tablespoons balsamic vinegar

Method

1 Put the turkey, zucchini, sage, white pepper, fennel and eggwhite in a bowl and mix until well combined. Divide the mixture in half and shape into two patties. Transfer to a plate, cover with plastic wrap and refrigerate for 30 minutes.

2 Meanwhile, to make the relish, combine the onion, fennel, apple and vinegar in a saucepan. Cover and cook over medium–low heat, stirring occasionally, for 20 minutes or until softened, adding 1 tablespoon of water if the mixture is becoming too dry. Spoon into a bowl and leave to cool for 15 minutes.

3 Preheat a barbecue plate or grill to medium–high. Spray the turkey patties with olive oil and cook for 4–5 minutes on both sides or until browned and cooked through.

4 Meanwhile, slice the bread rolls in half horizontally. Lightly spray the cut sides with olive oil and cook on the barbecue grill, cut side down, for 2–3 minutes or until lightly toasted.

5 To assemble the burgers, arrange the lettuce on the bases of the rolls. Add the turkey patties, relish, tomato, cucumber and some freshly ground black pepper. Replace the tops of the rolls and serve.

Serves 2
Preparation 15 minutes + 30 minutes chilling
Cooking 30 minutes

Nutrition	Per serve
Energy (kJ)	1680
Protein (g)	34
Carbohydrate (g)	44
Starches (g)	25
Sugars (g)	19
Exchanges	3
Portions	4.5
GI	Medium
GL	Medium
Protein:carbohydrate ratio	0.77
Fat (g)	7
Saturated fat (g)	1
Unsaturated fat (g)	6
Saturated:unsaturated ratio	0.17
Fibre (g)	11
Sodium (mg)	670
Potassium (mg)	1290
Sodium:potassium ratio	0.52
Gluten free?	No

notes

Refrigerate any left-over relish in a sealed container for up to a week. Make a double batch of patties and freeze the uncooked patties in resealable plastic bags for up to 3 months.

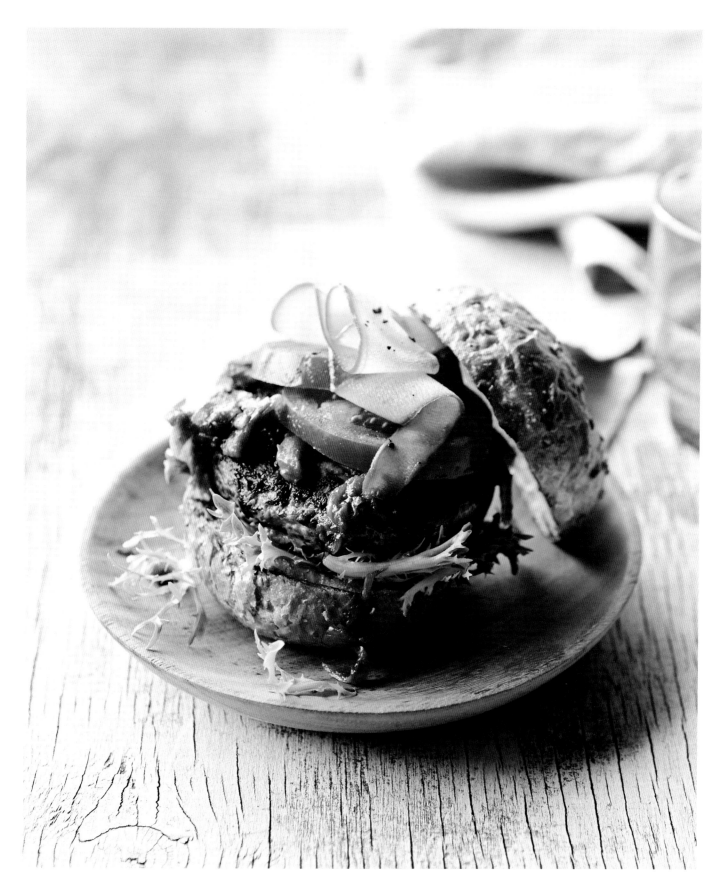

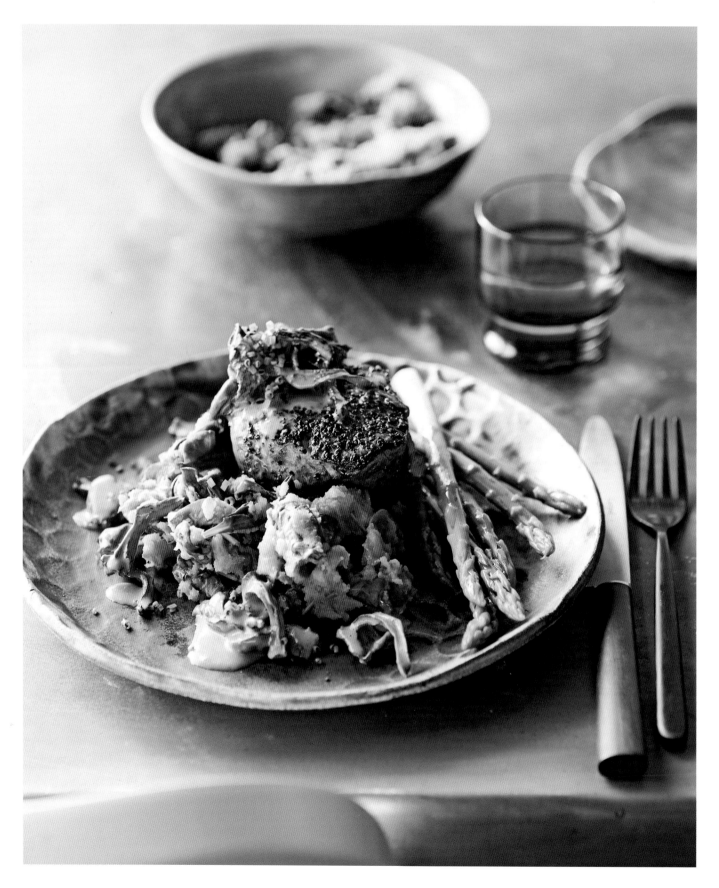

BEEF *with* SWEET POTATO MASH *and* WILD MUSHROOM SAUCE

For a rich, full-bodied, earthy flavour, use only dried porcini mushrooms. Alternatively, use any combination of fresh mushrooms. Mushrooms are packed with B-group vitamins and potassium.

Ingredients

25 g (1 oz) dried wild mushrooms

250 ml (9 fl oz/1 cup) boiling water

300 g (10½ oz) orange sweet potato, roughly chopped

60 g (2¼ oz/1⅓ cups) baby English spinach leaves

2 tablespoons snipped chives, plus extra to serve

olive oil spray

250 g (9 oz) button mushrooms, sliced

60 ml (2 fl oz/¼ cup) red wine

2 tablespoons reduced-fat cooking cream

1 teaspoon cracked black pepper

2 x 150 g (5½ oz) eye fillet steaks

200 g (7 oz) asparagus, steamed

Method

1 Put the dried mushrooms in a heatproof bowl, pour in the boiling water and soak for 30 minutes. Drain the mushrooms, reserving 125 ml (4 fl oz/½ cup) of the soaking liquid.

2 Cook the sweet potato in a saucepan of boiling water for 8–10 minutes or until soft. Drain and return to the pan, then roughly mash and stir in the spinach and chives. Cover and set aside until needed.

3 Meanwhile, spray a large frying pan with olive oil and place over medium–high heat. Cook the button mushrooms, stirring occasionally, for 5 minutes or until they start to release their juices. Add the wild mushrooms and red wine, and cook for 2 minutes or until the wine has reduced by half. Pour in the reserved soaking liquid and the cream, then reduce the heat to low and simmer, stirring occasionally, for 5 minutes or until the sauce has thickened and reduced by half.

4 Rub the pepper over the steaks. Spray a small frying pan with olive oil and place over medium–high heat. Cook the steaks for 2–3 minutes on each side or until browned and done to your liking.

5 Spoon the sweet potato mash onto two plates and top with the steaks and the mushroom sauce. Serve with the extra chives and asparagus.

Serves 2
Preparation 20 minutes +
30 minutes soaking
Cooking 20 minutes

Nutrition	Per serve
Energy (kJ)	1860
Protein (g)	43
Carbohydrate (g)	26
Starches (g)	15
Sugars (g)	11
Exchanges	1.5
Portions	2.5
GI	Medium
GL	Low
Protein:carbohydrate ratio	1.65
Fat (g)	14
Saturated fat (g)	7
Unsaturated fat (g)	7
Saturated:unsaturated ratio	1
Fibre (g)	9
Sodium (mg)	120
Potassium (mg)	1890
Sodium:potassium ratio	0.06
Gluten free?	Yes

note

The cooking time for the fillet steaks will vary depending on the thickness of the cut.

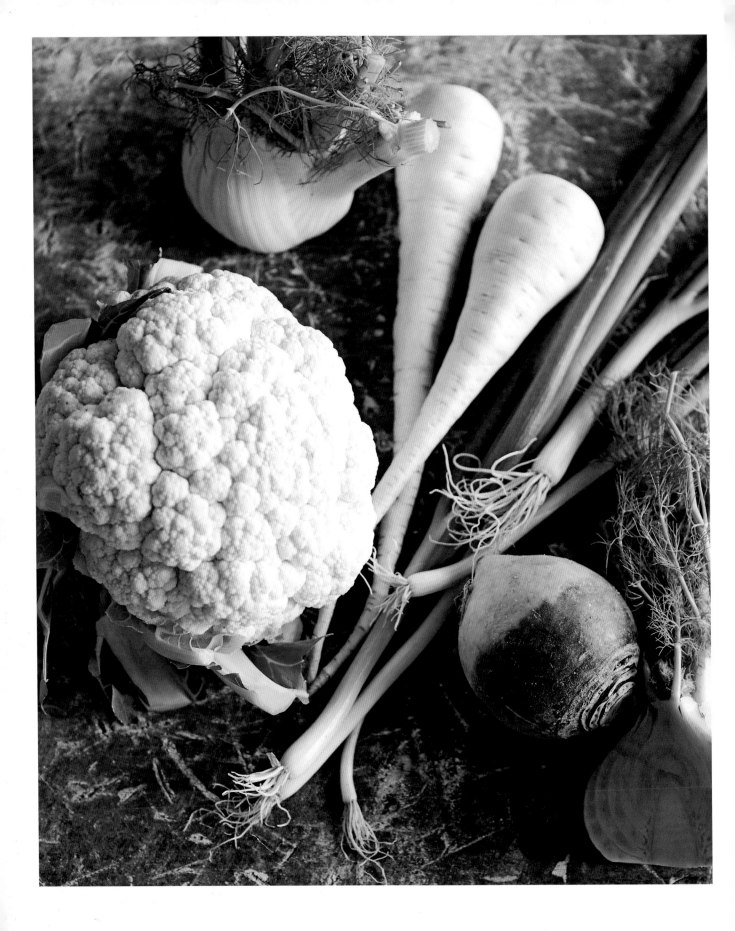

Chapter Four

VEGETARIAN DISHES

ROASTED BEETROOT, LENTIL *and* GOAT'S CHEESE SALAD

Puy lentils are tiny French blue-green lentils, which hold their shape when cooked. They have a nutty flavour and are a very good source of protein, dietary fibre and carbohydrates.

Ingredients

2 large beetroot (beets), peeled and cut into wedges

60 ml (2 fl oz/¼ cup) red wine vinegar

1 tablespoon honey

2 figs, quartered

210 g (7½ oz/1 cup) puy lentils or tiny blue-green lentils

olive oil spray

250 g (9 oz) Tuscan cabbage (cavolo nero), trimmed and halved

2 tablespoons fresh orange juice

1 teaspoon orange blossom water

60 g (2¼ oz) goat's cheese, crumbled

50 g (1¾ oz) chopped walnuts, toasted

1 small handful chives, snipped

Method

1 Preheat the oven to 180°C (350°F). Line a large baking tray with baking paper. Put the beetroot in a bowl and toss with half the vinegar and the honey. Spread the beetroot on the baking tray and roast for 20–25 minutes or until tender. Transfer the cooked beetroot to a plate, add the figs to the tray and roast for 5–6 minutes or until they start to soften. Transfer to the plate to cool.

2 Put the lentils and 750 ml (26 fl oz/3 cups) water in a saucepan. Bring to the boil over high heat, then reduce the heat and simmer for 20 minutes or until the lentils are tender. Drain and set aside.

3 Spray a large non-stick frying pan with olive oil and place over high heat. Cook the cabbage for 1–2 minutes or until just wilted. Add the remaining vinegar, the orange juice and orange blossom water, and stir to combine.

4 Arrange the cabbage, lentils, beetroot and figs on a platter. Top with the goat's cheese, walnuts and chives. Serve drizzled with the pan juices.

Serves 4
Preparation 20 minutes
Cooking 55 minutes

Nutrition	Per serve
Energy (kJ)	1450
Protein (g)	19
Carbohydrate (g)	34
Starches (g)	19
Sugars (g)	15
Exchanges	2.5
Portions	3.5
GI	Low
GL	Low
Protein:carbohydrate ratio	0.56
Fat (g)	13
Saturated fat (g)	2
Unsaturated fat (g)	11
Saturated:unsaturated ratio	0.18
Fibre (g)	12
Sodium (mg)	110
Potassium (mg)	920
Sodium:potassium ratio	0.12
Gluten free?	Yes

notes

To toast the walnuts, spread them on a baking tray and add them to the oven for 8–10 minutes while the beetroot is roasting. If figs are not in season, use pears instead. If puy lentils are unavailable, substitute them with green lentils.

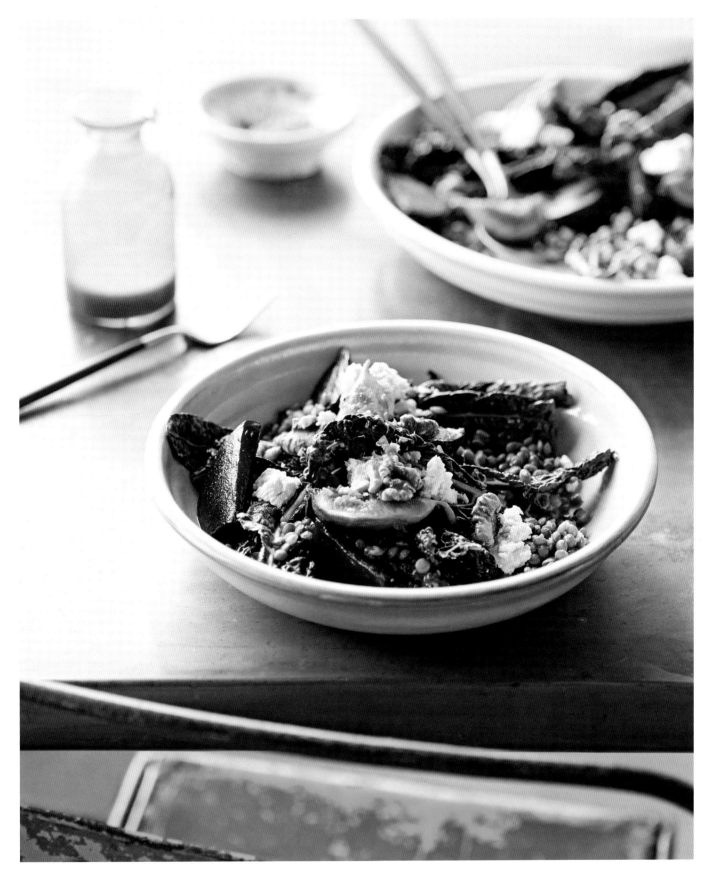

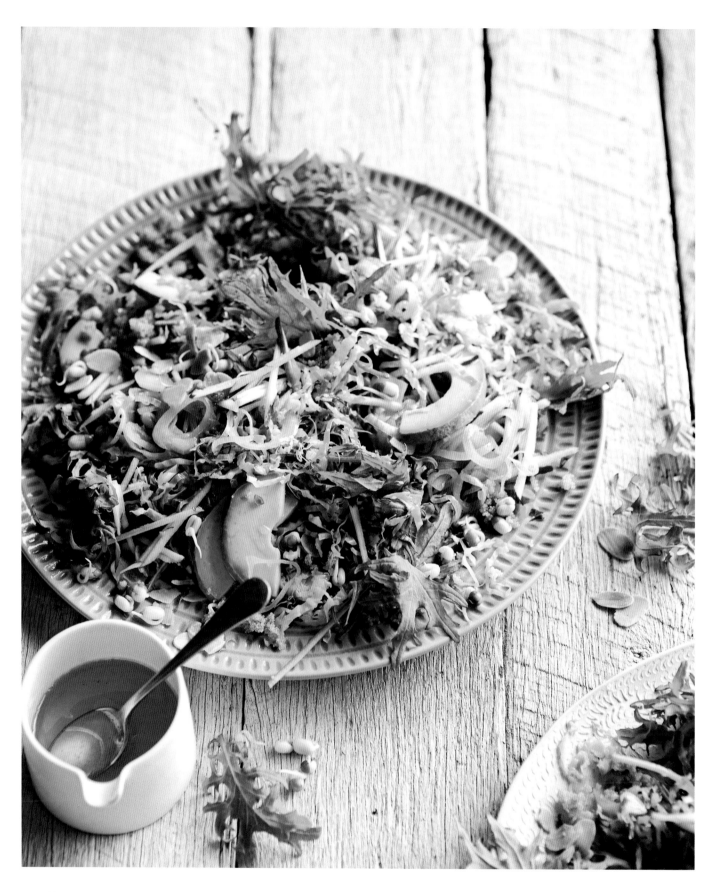

BRUSSELS SPROUT, KALE *and* AMARANTH SALAD

Amaranth is known as a super grain of the Aztecs. It has a nutty flavour and the seeds are rich in protein. They are a source of dietary fibre, magnesium and calcium, and even contain iron.

Ingredients

100 g (3½ oz/½ cup) amaranth
olive oil spray
2 French shallots, sliced
250 g (9 oz) brussels sprouts, shredded
120 g (4¼ oz) baby kale leaves
1 red apple, coarsely grated
1 avocado, sliced
100 g (3½ oz) mung bean sprouts
60 ml (2 fl oz/¼ cup) apple cider vinegar
1 tablespoon macadamia oil
2 tablespoons flaked almonds, toasted

Method

1 Put the amaranth and 750 ml (26 fl oz/3 cups) water in a saucepan. Bring to the boil over high heat, then reduce the heat, cover and simmer for 20–25 minutes or until the amaranth is tender but still retains a slight crunch. Drain and rinse to remove the excess starch. Spread the amaranth over a large baking tray and set aside to cool for 15 minutes.

2 Spray a large non-stick frying pan with olive oil and place over high heat. Cook the shallot slices, stirring, for 2 minutes or until softened. Add the brussels sprouts and stir for 1–2 minutes or until they are vibrant in colour and just starting to wilt.

3 Mix the amaranth, brussels sprouts, kale, apple, avocado and mung beans together in a large bowl.

4 Whisk the vinegar and macadamia oil in a small bowl. Pour over the salad and toss to combine. Serve with the almonds scattered over the top.

Serves 6
Preparation 20 minutes +
15 minutes cooling
Cooking 30 minutes

Nutrition	Per serve
Energy (kJ)	1045
Protein (g)	7
Carbohydrate (g)	17
Starches (g)	12
Sugars (g)	5
Exchanges	1
Portions	1.5
GI	Low
GL	Low
Protein:carbohydrate ratio	0.41
Fat (g)	16
Saturated fat (g)	3
Unsaturated fat (g)	13
Saturated:unsaturated ratio	0.23
Fibre (g)	6
Sodium (mg)	20
Potassium (mg)	590
Sodium:potassium ratio	0.03
Gluten free?	Yes

CURRIED CAULIFLOWER
and GREEN BEANS *with* SEEDS

Other vegetable varieties can also be used in this recipe – simply chop
up your favourites and add them to the wok with the beans.

Ingredients
1 tablespoon canola oil

1 large (1.5 kg/3 lb 5 oz)
    cauliflower, cut into
    small florets

1 red onion, sliced

40 g (1½ oz) piece fresh
    ginger, shredded

2 teaspoons cumin seeds

1 teaspoon yellow mustard
    seeds

1 teaspoon ground coriander

½ teaspoon garam masala

¼ teaspoon ground turmeric

400 g (14 oz) green beans,
    halved

1 long green chilli, thinly
    sliced

3 garlic cloves, sliced

1 tablespoon pepitas
    (pumpkin seeds)

1 teaspoon sesame seeds

1 teaspoon nigella seeds

1 large handful coriander
    (cilantro) leaves

200 g (7 oz/¾ cup) reduced-
    fat plain yoghurt

Method
1 Heat the canola oil in a large wok over high heat.
Stir-fry the cauliflower for 4–5 minutes or until
browned and starting to soften. Reduce the heat
to medium, add the onion, ginger, cumin seeds,
mustard seeds, ground coriander, garam masala
and turmeric, and stir-fry for 2 minutes or until
the spices are aromatic.

2 Add the green beans, chilli, garlic, pepitas,
sesame seeds, nigella seeds and 2 tablespoons
water to the wok. Stir-fry for 2 minutes or until
the beans have just softened.

3 Spoon the vegetable mixture onto a platter and
scatter the coriander leaves over the top. Serve
with the yoghurt.

Serves 4
Preparation 15 minutes
Cooking 10 minutes

Nutrition	Per serve
Energy (kJ)	1015
Protein (g)	16
Carbohydrate (g)	18
Starches (g)	4
Sugars (g)	14
Exchanges	1
Portions	2
GI	Low
GL	Low
Protein:carbohydrate ratio	0.89
Fat (g)	9
Saturated fat (g)	1
Unsaturated fat (g)	8
Saturated:unsaturated ratio	0.13
Fibre (g)	13
Sodium (mg)	100
Potassium (mg)	1790
Sodium:potassium ratio	0.06
Gluten free?	Yes

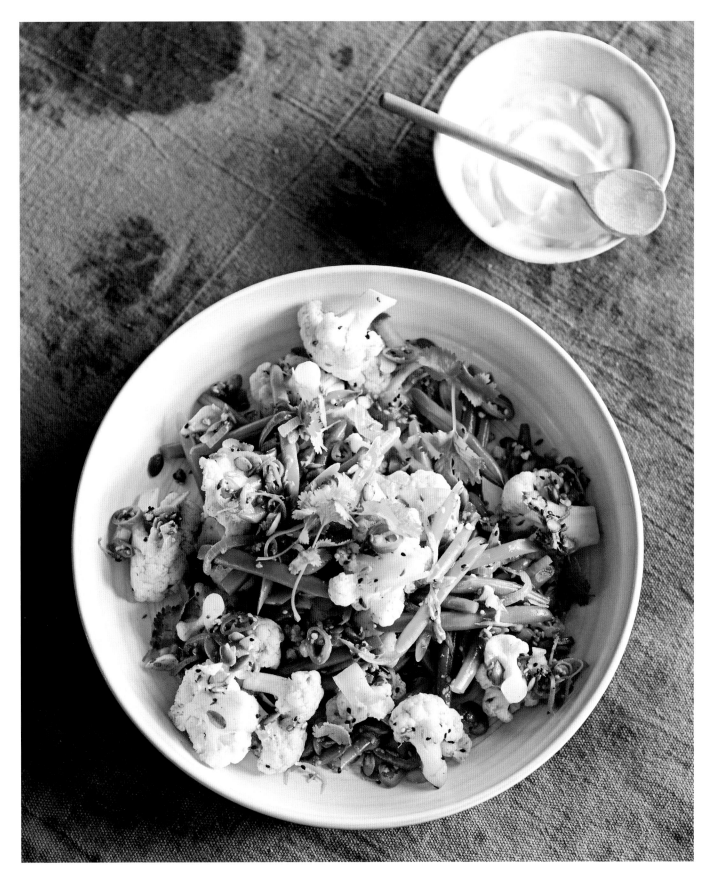

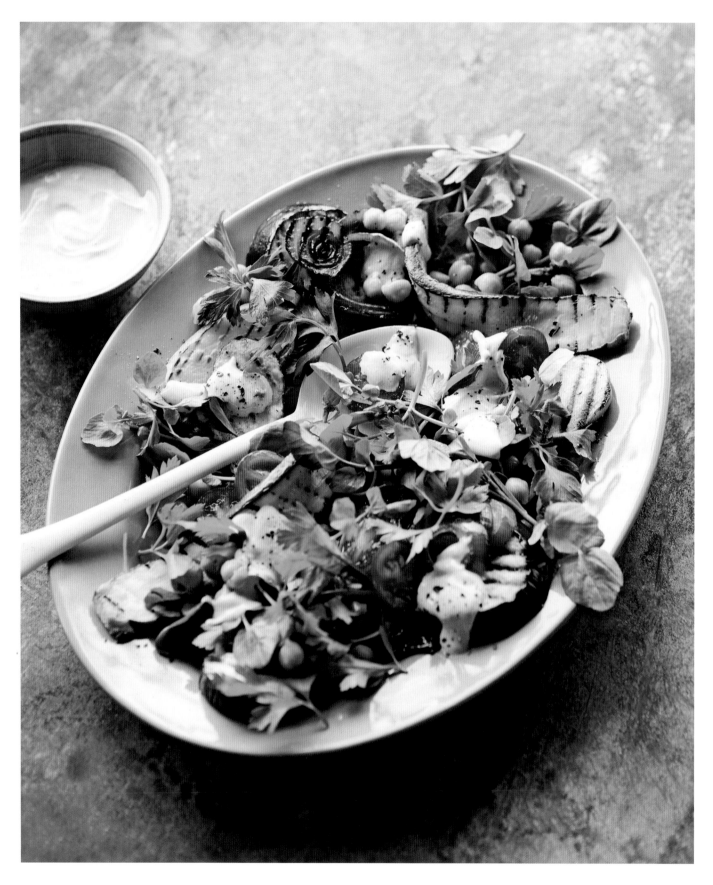

CHARGRILLED VEGETABLES
with TAHINI DRESSING

This dish is packed full of dietary fibre and potassium, and is moderate in low-GI carbohydrates. Sliced pumpkin (winter squash) or orange sweet potato also work well in this recipe.

Ingredients

1 large eggplant (aubergine), sliced

2 large zucchini (courgettes), sliced lengthways

2 large lower-GI potatoes, such as Carisma, sliced

1 red onion, sliced

olive oil spray

250 g (9 oz) cherry tomatoes, halved

1 small handful parsley leaves

400 g (14 oz) tinned no-added-salt chickpeas, rinsed and drained

120 g (4¼ oz) watercress sprigs

Tahini dressing

250 g (9 oz) fat-free plain yoghurt

2 tablespoons unhulled tahini

2 tablespoons lemon juice

Method

1 Heat a chargrill pan over medium–high heat. Lightly spray the eggplant, zucchini, potatoes and onion with olive oil. Cook the vegetables in batches for 2–3 minutes on each side or until golden and tender. Transfer to a plate until required.

2 To make the tahini dressing, combine the yoghurt, tahini and lemon juice in a small bowl and mix well.

3 Arrange the eggplant, zucchini, potatoes, onion, tomatoes, parsley, chickpeas and watercress sprigs on a platter. Dollop the tahini dressing over the salad, sprinkle with freshly ground black pepper and serve.

Serves 4
Preparation 25 minutes
Cooking 20 minutes

Nutrition	Per serve
Energy (kJ)	1400
Protein (g)	18
Carbohydrate (g)	35
Starches (g)	24
Sugars (g)	11
Exchanges	2.5
Portions	3.5
GI	Low
GL	Low
Protein:carbohydrate ratio	0.51
Fat (g)	10
Saturated fat (g)	1
Unsaturated fat (g)	9
Saturated:unsaturated ratio	0.11
Fibre (g)	14
Sodium (mg)	340
Potassium (mg)	1520
Sodium:potassium ratio	0.22
Gluten free?	Yes

note

Tahini is a paste made from sesame seeds. It is sold in both hulled and unhulled varieties. Choose the unhulled variety for more fibre. Stir it before using as the oil will settle on the surface.

POTATO *and* CAULIFLOWER MASALA DOSA

Dosa, or Thosai, originated in South India. It is traditionally a breakfast dish of a fermented crepe with a spiced potato filling. This full-flavoured, low-fat and high-fibre option includes dried spices for a healthy meal.

Ingredients

300 g (10½ oz) lower-GI potatoes, such as Carisma, cut into small cubes

350 g (12 oz) cauliflower, cut into small florets

2 tablespoons curry leaves, plus extra to serve

olive oil spray

1 brown onion, sliced

2 long green chillies, sliced, plus extra to serve

30 g (1 oz) piece fresh ginger, finely grated

2 teaspoons yellow mustard seeds

1 teaspoon cumin seeds

½ teaspoon ground turmeric

150 g (5½ oz) reduced-fat plain yoghurt

coriander (cilantro) sprigs, to serve

Dosa

60 g (2¼ oz/½ cup) chickpea flour (besan)

75 g (2½ oz/½ cup) wholemeal plain (wholewheat all-purpose) flour

45 g (1½ oz/¼ cup) rice flour

1 small handful coriander (cilantro) leaves, finely chopped

olive oil spray

Method

1 Put the potatoes in a saucepan of water and bring to the boil over high heat. Reduce the heat and cook for 8 minutes. Add the cauliflower and cook for a further 2–3 minutes or until the cauliflower is tender and the potatoes are soft when tested with a knife. Drain the vegetables and set aside.

2 Lightly spray the extra curry leaves with olive oil. Cook in a large non-stick frying pan over medium heat for 1–2 minutes or until crisp. Remove from the pan and set aside.

3 Spray the frying pan with olive oil and place over medium heat. Add the onion and cook, stirring, for 2–3 minutes or until softened. Add the remaining curry leaves, chillies, ginger, mustard seeds, cumin seeds and turmeric. Cook, stirring, for 2–3 minutes or until aromatic. Add the potatoes, cauliflower and 60 ml (2 fl oz/¼ cup) water. Stir for 1 minute or until combined and the potatoes are slightly mashed. Cover and keep warm while you cook the dosa.

4 To make the dosa, combine the flours with 310 ml (10¾ fl oz/1¼ cups) water and whisk to make a runny batter. Stir in the coriander. Spray a large frying pan with olive oil and place over medium heat. Add a quarter of the batter to the pan, tilting and swirling to make a thin round. Cook for 2 minutes, then turn over and cook for 1 minute or until golden. Transfer to a plate and repeat with the remaining batter to make four dosa in total.

5 Divide the potato mixture among the dosa, fold over and top with the yoghurt, coriander sprigs, extra chilli and fried curry leaves. Sprinkle with freshly ground black pepper and serve.

Serves 4
Preparation 20 minutes
Cooking 35 minutes

Nutrition	Per serve
Energy (kJ)	1225
Protein (g)	13
Carbohydrate (g)	48
Starches (g)	39
Sugars (g)	9
Exchanges	3
Portions	5
GI	Medium
GL	Low
Protein:carbohydrate ratio	0.27
Fat (g)	4
Saturated fat (g)	1
Unsaturated fat (g)	3
Saturated:unsaturated ratio	0.33
Fibre (g)	8
Sodium (mg)	50
Potassium (mg)	1070
Sodium:potassium ratio	0.05
Gluten free?	No

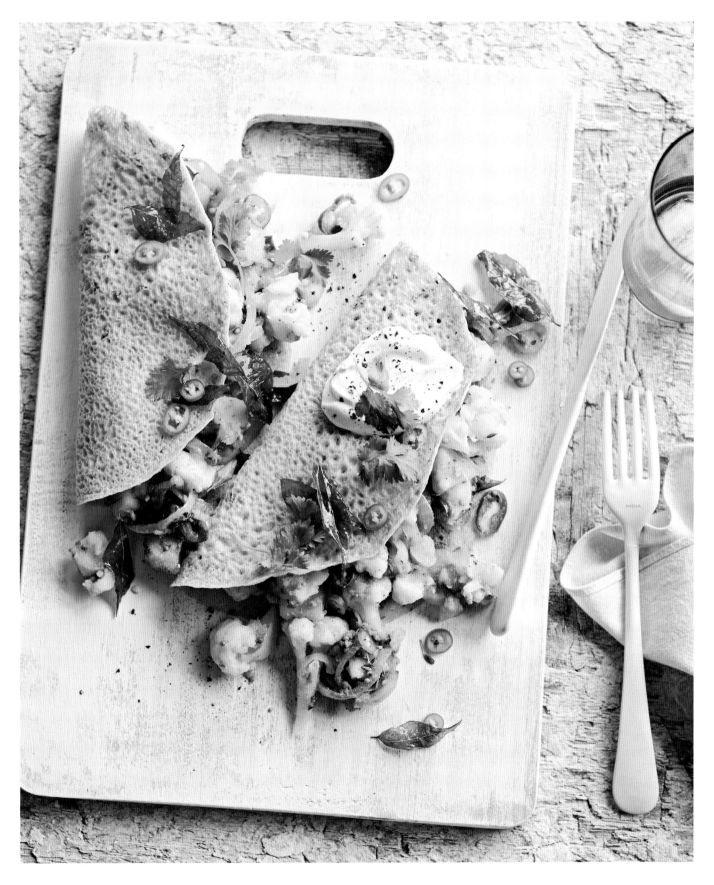

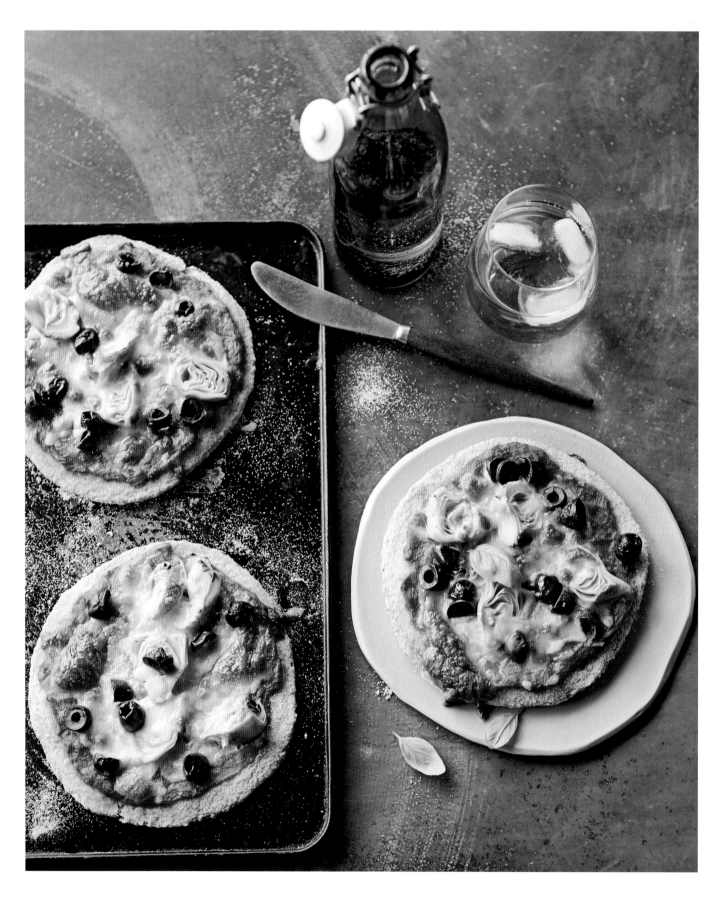

TOMATO, MOZZARELLA *and* OLIVE QUINOA PIZZAS

Quinoa has a light, nutty texture with a slight crunch. It is naturally low in fat, high in protein and fibre, and is gluten free. The quinoa will give the pizza bases a lovely crisp texture.

Ingredients

50 g (1¾ oz/¼ cup) quinoa, rinsed

2 teaspoons instant dried yeast

150 g (5½ oz/1 cup) wholemeal plain (whole-wheat all-purpose) flour

75 g (2½ oz/½ cup) stone-ground plain (all-purpose) flour

semolina, for sprinkling

140 g (5 oz) artichoke hearts in brine, rinsed and halved

100 g (3½ oz) reduced-fat grated mozzarella cheese

60 g (2¼ oz/⅓ cup) black olives, halved

1 handful basil leaves

200 g (7 oz) baby English spinach leaves

250 g (9 oz) baby roma (plum) tomatoes, halved

1 small Lebanese (short) cucumber, thinly sliced

2 tablespoons balsamic vinegar

Tomato sauce

2 teaspoons olive oil

1 brown onion, finely chopped

2 garlic cloves, crushed

500 g (1 lb 2 oz) ripe tomatoes, finely chopped

Method

1 Put the quinoa and 125 ml (4 fl oz/½ cup) water in a saucepan and bring to the boil. Reduce the heat, cover and simmer for 10–12 minutes or until all the liquid has evaporated. Transfer to a bowl to cool.

2 Stir the yeast into 185 ml (6 fl oz/¾ cup) tepid water until the yeast has dissolved. Combine the quinoa and flours in a large bowl. Make a well in the centre, add the yeast mixture and mix to a soft dough. Turn the dough out onto a lightly floured surface and knead for 10 minutes or until smooth and elastic. Return the dough to the lightly oiled bowl, cover with a tea towel (dish towel) and rest in a warm place for 1 hour or until doubled in size.

3 To make the sauce, heat the oil in a saucepan over medium heat. Cook the onion, stirring, for 4 minutes or until softened. Add the garlic and stir for 1 minute. Add the tomatoes, reduce the heat to low, cover and simmer, stirring occasionally, for 15 minutes or until the sauce has thickened. Remove the lid and cook for 5 minutes or until reduced by two-thirds. Set aside to cool, then purée using a stick blender.

4 Preheat the oven to 220°C (425°F). Sprinkle two large baking trays with semolina. Divide the dough into four portions and roll each on a lightly floured surface into a 20 cm (8 inch) round, about 5 mm (¼ inch) thick. Place on the prepared trays.

5 Spread the tomato sauce over the bases, then top with the artichokes, mozzarella and olives. Bake the pizzas for 18–20 minutes or until crisp and golden. Top with the basil leaves and cut into wedges.

6 Drizzle the spinach, tomatoes and cucumber with the vinegar and serve with the pizzas.

Serves 4

Preparation 20 minutes + 1 hour resting

Cooking 1 hour

Nutrition	Per serve
Energy (kJ)	1790
Protein (g)	21
Carbohydrate (g)	58
Starches (g)	48
Sugars (g)	10
Exchanges	4
Portions	6
GI	Low
GL	High
Protein:carbohydrate ratio	0.36
Fat (g)	9.5
Saturated fat (g)	3
Unsaturated fat (g)	6.5
Saturated:unsaturated ratio	0.46
Fibre (g)	11
Sodium (mg)	270
Potassium (mg)	1150
Sodium:potassium ratio	0.23
Gluten free?	No

PASTA *with* CAPSICUM *and* ROCKET

Use rice pasta to make this colourful dish gluten free. For a non-vegetarian option, add some sliced poached chicken breast.

Ingredients

olive oil spray

1 red onion, thickly sliced

1 red capsicum (pepper), thickly sliced

1 yellow capsicum (pepper), thickly sliced

2 tablespoons white wine vinegar

300 g (10½ oz) wholemeal (whole-wheat) spiral pasta

65 g (2¼ oz/¼ cup) reduced-fat sour cream

80 g (2¾ oz) baby rocket (arugula)

1 large handful basil leaves, shredded

200 g (7 oz) mixed salad leaves

1 tablespoon white balsamic vinegar

Method

1 Spray a large non-stick frying pan with olive oil, place over medium–high heat and cook the onion and capsicums for 6–8 minutes or until tender. Add the white wine vinegar, reduce the heat to low and cook for 2 minutes or until the vegetables are soft. Remove from the heat and set aside.

2 Cook the pasta in a large saucepan of boiling water over high heat until al dente. Drain the pasta, reserving 185 ml (6 fl oz/¾ cup) of the water.

3 Return the pasta to the pan with the reserved water and the sour cream. Add the rocket and stir until just wilted. Stir in the capsicum mixture until well combined.

4 Sprinkle the pasta with the shredded basil and freshly ground black pepper. Drizzle the salad leaves with the balsamic vinegar and serve with the pasta.

Serves 4
Preparation 20 minutes
Cooking 25 minutes

Nutrition	Per serve
Energy (kJ)	1350
Protein (g)	12
Carbohydrate (g)	50
Starches (g)	45
Sugars (g)	5
Exchanges	3.5
Portions	5
GI	Low
GL	Low
Protein:carbohydrate ratio	0.24
Fat (g)	6
Saturated fat (g)	2
Unsaturated fat (g)	4
Saturated:unsaturated ratio	0.5
Fibre (g)	9
Sodium (mg)	40
Potassium (mg)	560
Sodium:potassium ratio	0.07
Gluten free?	No

note

Cool and refrigerate the finished dish to serve as a cold pasta salad.

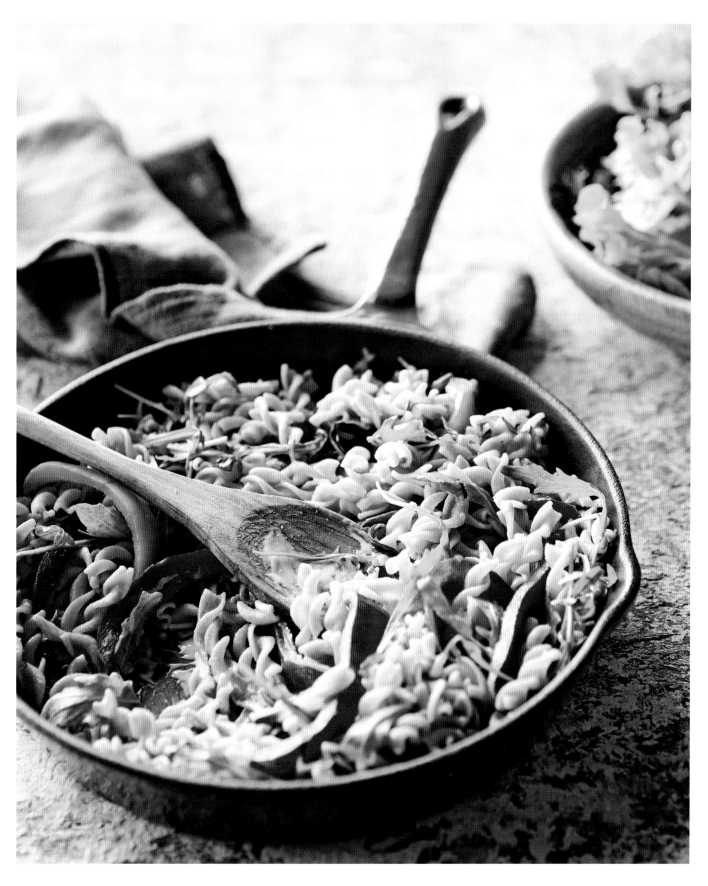

FRESH SPINACH *and* BASIL KAMUT PASTA

Kamut flour contains more protein and minerals than other flours, which makes this fresh pasta a great standby for people with diabetes. Simply toss the hot pasta with your favourite pasta sauce for a delicious meal.

Ingredients

300 g (10½ oz) organic kamut flour
60 g (2¼ oz/1⅓ cups) baby English spinach leaves
1 large handful basil leaves
2 teaspoons cracked black pepper
2 teaspoons finely grated lemon zest
3 eggs
95 g (3¼ oz/½ cup) semolina

Method

1 Put the kamut flour, spinach, basil, pepper and lemon zest in the bowl of a food processor. Blend for 30 seconds or until the spinach and basil are chopped and the ingredients are combined. Add the eggs and blend for 30 seconds or until the mixture resembles coarse breadcrumbs.

2 Turn the mixture out onto a clean work surface and bring it together with your hands. Shape the dough into a flattened disc, then wrap it in plastic wrap and refrigerate for 30 minutes.

3 Divide the dough into four portions. Sprinkle a work surface and the pasta with the semolina. Use a pasta machine or rolling pin to roll out the dough as thinly as possible, then cut the dough into 1 cm (½ inch) strips.

4 Bring a large saucepan of water to the boil over high heat. Add the pasta strips and cook, stirring, for 3–4 minutes or until al dente. Drain the pasta and serve with a few spoonfuls of Roasted tomato and capsicum relish (page 84), Rocket and basil pesto (page 85), or another sauce of your choice.

Serves 6
Preparation 30 minutes +
30 minutes chilling
Cooking 5 minutes

Nutrition	Per serve
Energy (kJ)	1120
Protein (g)	13
Carbohydrate (g)	41
Starches (g)	40
Sugars (g)	1
Exchanges	2.5
Portions	4
GI	Low
GL	Low
Protein:carbohydrate ratio	0.32
Fat (g)	4.5
Saturated fat (g)	1
Unsaturated fat (g)	3.5
Saturated:unsaturated ratio	0.29
Fibre (g)	6.5
Sodium (mg)	45
Potassium (mg)	320
Sodium:potassium ratio	0.14
Gluten free?	No

note

Kamut is an ancient variety of wheat from the Persian province of Khorasan. It is known for its buttery, nutty flavour. Look for kamut flour in health food stores and speciality grocery stores.

CHILLI *and* PARMESAN PASTA

Fresh pasta with a simple topping makes a quick light meal. This recipe uses the Fresh spinach and basil kamut pasta (see opposite), but you can also use any other fresh or dried pasta.

Ingredients

1 quantity Fresh spinach and basil kamut pasta (opposite page), cooked and drained

2 tablespoons extra virgin olive oil

1 long red chilli, frozen

20 g (¾ oz) shaved parmesan cheese

small basil leaves, to serve

Method

1 Return the hot pasta to the cooking pan and drizzle with the olive oil.

2 Divide the pasta among six serving bowls. Using a microplane, grate the frozen chilli over the top. Serve the pasta sprinkled with the parmesan shavings and basil leaves.

Serves 6
Preparation 10 minutes
Cooking Nil

Nutrition	Per serve
Energy (kJ)	1410
Protein (g)	14
Carbohydrate (g)	41
Starches (g)	40
Sugars (g)	1
Exchanges	2.5
Portions	4
GI	Low
GL	Low
Protein:carbohydrate ratio	0.34
Fat (g)	11
Saturated fat (g)	2.5
Unsaturated fat (g)	8.5
Saturated:unsaturated ratio	0.29
Fibre (g)	7
Sodium (mg)	90
Potassium (mg)	350
Sodium:potassium ratio	0.26
Gluten free?	No

note

The nutrition values for this recipe have been calculated using the Fresh spinach and basil kamut pasta. If you use a different pasta, the values will vary.

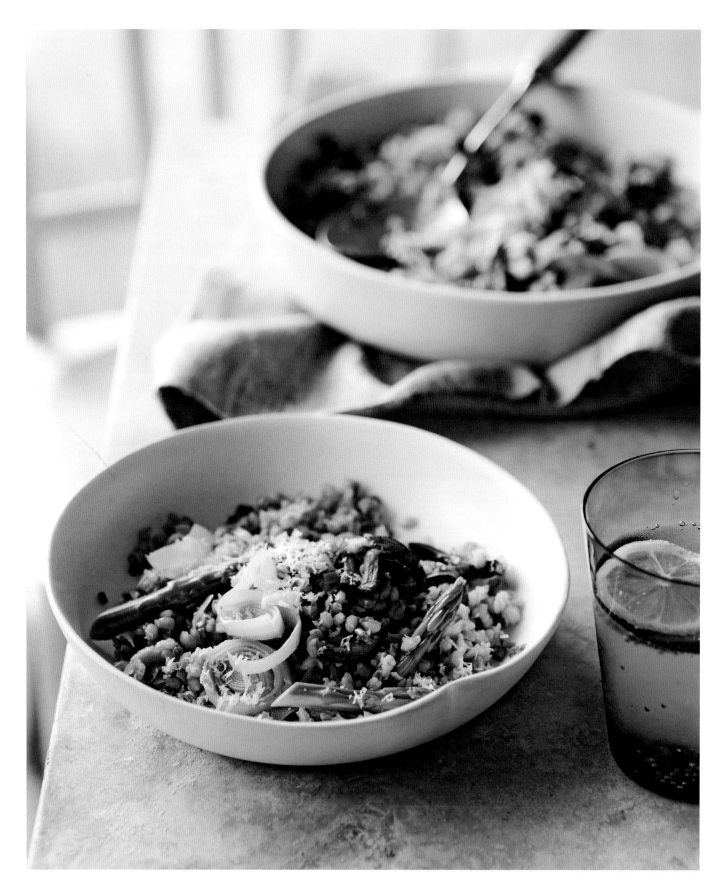

PEARL BARLEY, LEEK *and* MUSHROOM RISOTTO

Barley is one of the oldest cereal grains. It has a low GI value and is rich in magnesium.

Ingredients

2 leeks
400 g (14 oz) asparagus
1 brown onion, roughly chopped
2 celery stalks, chopped
2 carrots, chopped
4 thyme sprigs
4 parsley stems
bouquet garni
10 black peppercorns
1 tablespoon olive oil
250 g (9 oz) portobello mushrooms, sliced
80 ml (2½ fl oz/⅓ cup) dry white wine
200 g (7 oz/1 cup) pearl barley, rinsed
25 g (1 oz/¼ cup) finely grated parmesan cheese
2 tablespoons snipped chives

Method

1 Roughly chop the green parts of the leeks and thinly slice the white parts. Trim the asparagus, reserving the trimmings for the stock. Cut the spears into 4 cm (1½ inch) lengths.

2 Put the green parts of the leeks, the asparagus trimmings, onion, celery, carrots, thyme, parsley, bouquet garni and peppercorns in a stockpot or very large saucepan. Pour in 1.5 litres (52 fl oz/ 6 cups) water, cover and simmer the stock over low heat for 45 minutes. Strain through a piece of muslin (cheesecloth), discarding the vegetables. Measure out 750 ml (26 fl oz/3 cups) of the stock.

3 Heat a large saucepan over medium heat. Add the oil and cook the sliced leeks for 2 minutes or until softened. Add the mushrooms and cook, stirring, for 3–4 minutes or until tender.

4 Pour the wine into the mushroom mixture and stir for 1 minute or until the wine has evaporated. Add the barley and 250 ml (9 fl oz/1 cup) of the stock and stir until the stock has been absorbed. Continue adding the stock gradually, stirring occasionally, for 25–30 minutes or until all the stock has been absorbed. Add the asparagus pieces for the last 2–3 minutes of cooking.

5 Spoon the risotto into serving bowls and serve topped with the parmesan and chives.

Serves 4
Preparation 45 minutes
Cooking 1 hour 25 minutes

Nutrition	Per serve
Energy (kJ)	1355
Protein (g)	13
Carbohydrate (g)	39
Starches (g)	32
Sugars (g)	7
Exchanges	2.5
Portions	4
GI	Low
GL	Low
Protein:carbohydrate ratio	0.33
Fat (g)	8
Saturated fat (g)	2
Unsaturated fat (g)	6
Saturated:unsaturated ratio	0.33
Fibre (g)	13
Sodium (mg)	160
Potassium (mg)	1020
Sodium:potassium ratio	0.16
Gluten free?	No

notes

Freeze any left-over stock for other recipes. A bouquet garni is a bundle of herbs tied together with string, usually containing thyme, parsley and bay leaves. They are available with the fresh herbs in the fruit and vegetable section or in dried form in the herb aisle of supermarkets.

CARAMELISED ONION, PEAR *and* WALNUT TART

Onions contain the antioxidant quercetin, which can act as a natural anti-inflammatory. Take time to slowly cook the onions for a rich, sweet and deeply coloured result.

Ingredients

olive oil spray

4 large brown onions, sliced into rings

80 ml (2½ fl oz/⅓ cup) balsamic vinegar

1½ sheets (240 g/8½ oz) reduced-fat puff pastry, just thawed

150 g (5½ oz) baby roma (plum) tomatoes, halved

1 baby fennel bulb, thinly sliced

30 g (1 oz/¼ cup) walnuts, chopped

80 g (2¾ oz) baby rocket (arugula)

1 small pear, thinly sliced

100 g (3½ oz) low-fat cottage cheese

Method

1 Spray a large saucepan with olive oil and place over medium–low heat. Cook the onions, stirring, for 10 minutes or until softened. Reduce the heat and pour in 60 ml (2 fl oz/¼ cup) of the vinegar. Cover and cook the onions, stirring occasionally, for 20 minutes or until soft and caramelised. Set aside to cool for 15 minutes.

2 Preheat the oven to 200°C (400°F). Spray an 11 x 34 cm (4¼ x 13½ inch) loose-based fluted flan (tart) tin with olive oil. Line the tin with the pastry, pressing the overlapping pastry with your fingertips to seal it, and trim the edges. Spread the caramelised onion over the pastry. Bake for 20 minutes or until the pastry is puffed and golden. Add the tomato halves to a baking tray, spray with olive oil and cook with the tart for the last 10 minutes or until the tomatoes are just softened. Set aside to cool for 15 minutes.

3 Scatter a quarter of the fennel slices, the tomato halves, walnuts and a few of the rocket leaves over the tart. Mix the pear with the remaining fennel and rocket, and drizzle with the remaining vinegar. Serve the tart and salad with the cottage cheese.

Serves 6
Preparation 15 minutes +
15 minutes cooling
Cooking 50 minutes

Nutrition	Per serve
Energy (kJ)	1015
Protein (g)	9
Carbohydrate (g)	29
Starches (g)	20
Sugars (g)	9
Exchanges	2
Portions	3
GI	Medium
GL	Low
Protein:carbohydrate ratio	0.31
Fat (g)	9
Saturated fat (g)	3
Unsaturated fat (g)	6
Saturated:unsaturated ratio	0.5
Fibre (g)	5
Sodium (mg)	200
Potassium (mg)	455
Sodium:potassium ratio	0.44
Gluten free?	No

notes

The caramelised onions can be prepared up to 2 days ahead. Bring them to room temperature before using. Chopped hazelnuts can be used instead of walnuts.

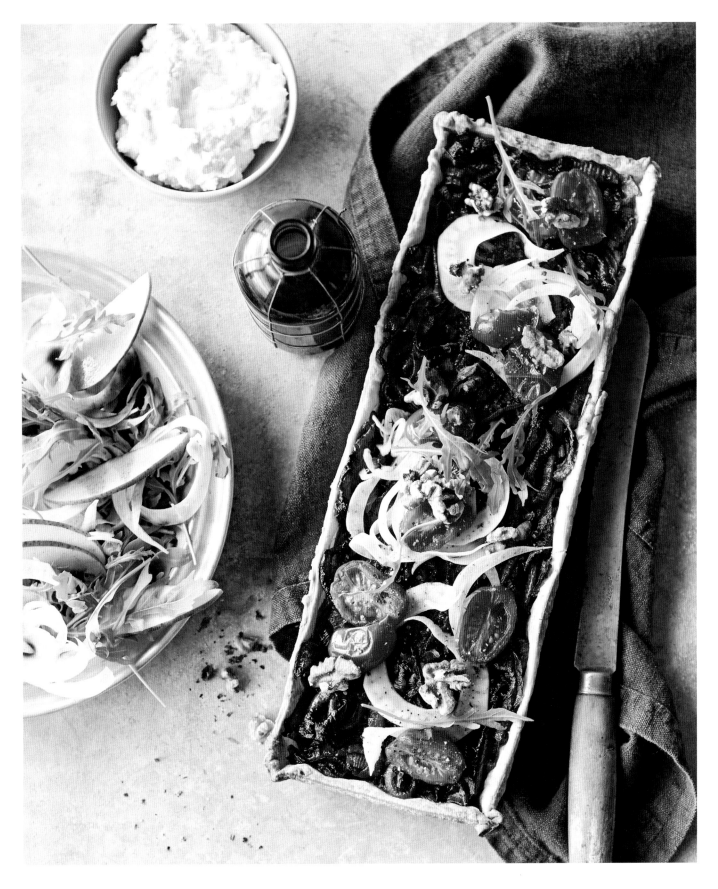

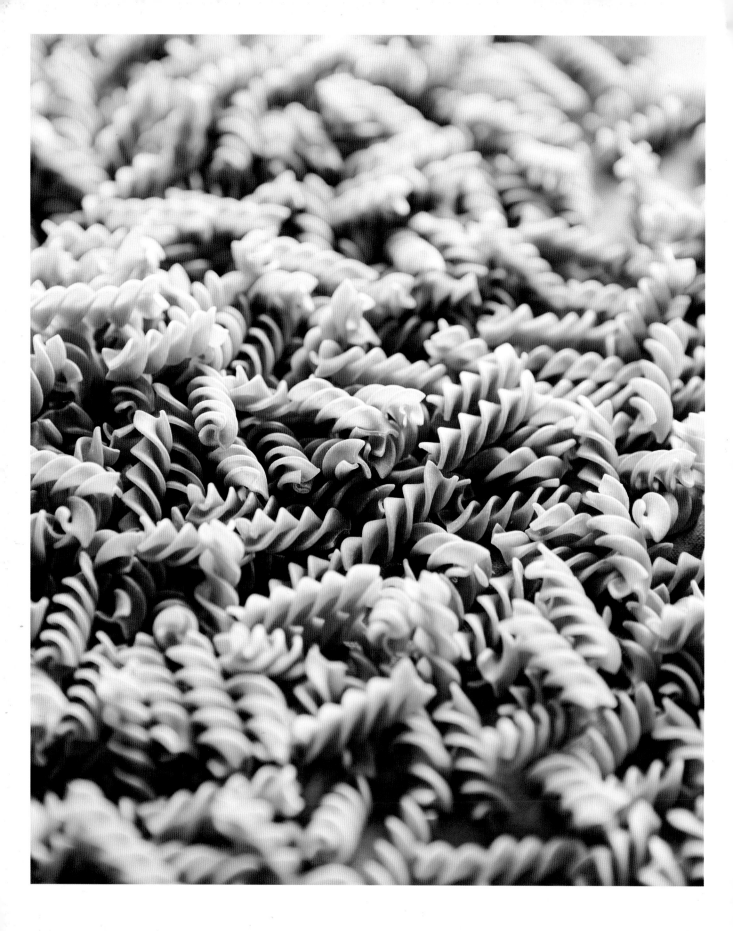

Chapter Five

MAIN MEALS

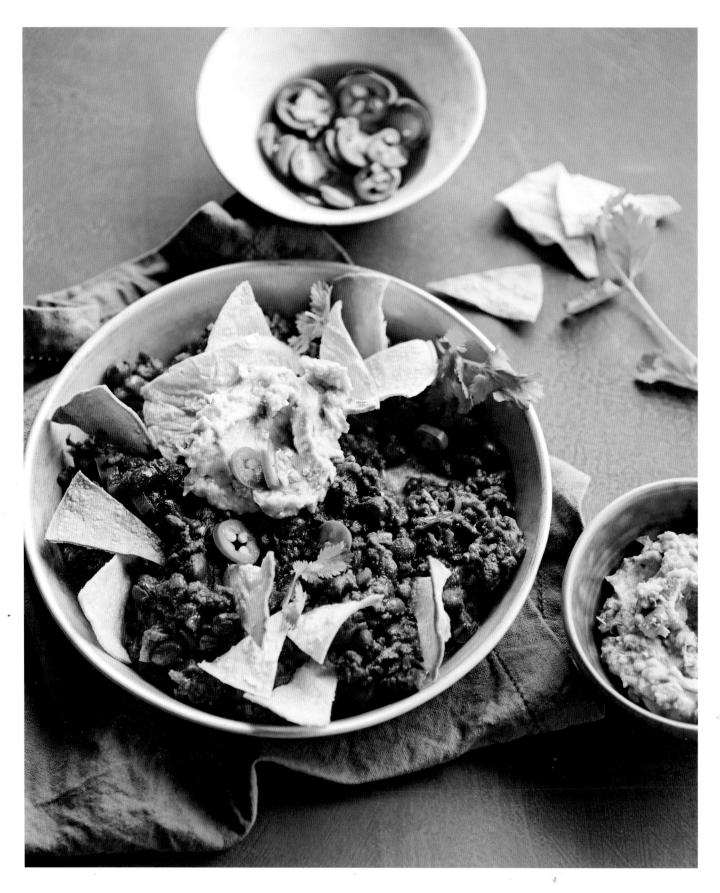

BEEF *and* BEAN NACHOS

Thanks to the kidney beans, this dish is moderate in low-GI carbohydrate and very high in dietary fibre and potassium. Make a double batch of the beef and bean mixture to freeze for another meal.

Ingredients

4 jalapeños, thinly sliced
2 tablespoons malt vinegar
4 x 26 g (1 oz) low-sodium white corn tortillas
olive oil spray
1 brown onion, finely chopped
2 celery stalks, finely chopped
1 green capsicum (pepper), finely chopped
300 g (10½ oz) extra-lean minced (ground) beef
1 tablespoon smoked paprika
2 teaspoons ground cumin
2 teaspoons dried oregano
400 g (14 oz) tinned diced tomatoes
800 g (1 lb 12 oz) tinned no-added-salt kidney beans, rinsed and drained
1 small avocado
2 teaspoons lemon juice
1 small handful coriander (cilantro) leaves, finely chopped, plus extra sprigs to serve

Method

1 Put the jalapeños in a small bowl with the vinegar and set aside to marinate.

2 Preheat the oven to 180°C (350°F). Lightly spray both sides of the tortillas with olive oil. Cut each tortilla into 10 wedges and arrange on a large baking tray. Bake, turning once, for 10–12 minutes or until golden and crisp. Set aside until needed.

3 While the tortilla crisps are cooking, spray a large saucepan with olive oil and place over medium heat. Add the onion and cook, stirring, for 2 minutes or until softened. Add the celery and capsicum, and stir for 6–7 minutes or until browned and softened. Add the beef and cook, stirring and breaking up any lumps, for 5 minutes or until browned.

4 Stir in the paprika, cumin and oregano, and cook for 2 minutes or until fragrant. Stir in the tomatoes and 185 ml (6 fl oz/¾ cup) water. Reduce the heat, cover and simmer for 25–30 minutes or until the sauce has thickened. Add the beans and cook for 10 minutes.

5 Meanwhile, mash the avocado with a fork, then stir in the lemon juice and chopped coriander. Season with freshly ground black pepper.

6 Spoon the beef and bean mixture into bowls and serve with the tortilla crisps, avocado, extra coriander and jalapeños.

Serves 4
Preparation 30 minutes
Cooking 1 hour

Nutrition	Per serve
Energy (kJ)	2850
Protein (g)	48
Carbohydrate (g)	51
Starches (g)	37
Sugars (g)	14
Exchanges	3.5
Portions	5
GI	Low
GL	Low
Protein:carbohydrate ratio	0.94
Fat (g)	24
Saturated fat (g)	6
Unsaturated fat (g)	18
Saturated:unsaturated ratio	0.33
Fibre (g)	28
Sodium (mg)	400
Potassium (mg)	1845
Sodium:potassium ratio	0.22
Gluten free?	Yes

note

Spice up the tortillas by sprinkling them with cayenne pepper before baking.

BOSTON BAKED BEANS *with* POACHED EGGS

Great northern beans are small white beans that are traditionally used to make baked beans. They are also sold as navy beans, haricot or white beans, and are available in health food stores and speciality delicatessens.

Ingredients

290 g (10¼ oz/1½ cups) dried great northern beans, soaked overnight
olive oil spray
1 large brown onion, finely chopped
2 garlic cloves, chopped
2 teaspoons mustard powder
1 tablespoon sweet paprika
2 teaspoons ground cumin
1 teaspoon dried oregano
800 g (1 lb 12 oz) tinned diced tomatoes
1 tablespoon pure maple syrup
2 dried bay leaves
200 g (7 oz) lean minced (ground) pork
½ teaspoon hickory liquid smoke (optional)
1 tablespoon white vinegar
6 eggs
chopped parsley leaves, to serve

Method

1 Drain and rinse the beans, place in a saucepan and cover with water. Bring to the boil, then reduce the heat and simmer for 40–45 minutes or until tender. Drain the beans, reserving 500 ml (17 fl oz/2 cups) of the water.

2 Spray a large flameproof casserole dish with olive oil and place over medium heat. Cook the onion, stirring, for 3–4 minutes or until softened. Add the garlic and stir for 1 minute, then add the mustard, paprika, cumin and oregano, and stir for 2 minutes or until fragrant. Stir in the tomatoes, beans, maple syrup, bay leaves and reserved water. Reduce the heat to low, cover and cook for 1¾ hours or until the beans are soft and the sauce has thickened.

3 Meanwhile, heat a small non-stick frying pan over medium–high heat. Add the pork and hickory liquid smoke (if using) and cook for 5–6 minutes or until the pork is golden and cooked.

4 Just before the beans are cooked, bring a small saucepan of water to the boil over high heat. Add the vinegar and stir the water in a circular motion. Reduce the heat to low, crack an egg into a small bowl and gently pour it into the swirling water. Repeat with another egg. Simmer for 2 minutes, then remove from the water with a slotted spoon. Cook the remaining eggs in the same way.

5 Serve the beans topped with the pork mixture and eggs, and scatter over the parsley.

Serves 6

Preparation 25 minutes + overnight soaking
Cooking 2 hours 40 minutes

Nutrition	Per serve
Energy (kJ)	1500
Protein (g)	28
Carbohydrate (g)	31
Starches (g)	21
Sugars (g)	10
Exchanges	2
Portions	3
GI	Low
GL	Low
Protein:carbohydrate ratio	0.9
Fat (g)	9
Saturated fat (g)	2
Unsaturated fat (g)	7
Saturated:unsaturated ratio	0.29
Fibre (g)	13
Sodium (mg)	195
Potassium (mg)	1450
Sodium:potassium ratio	0.13
Gluten free?	Yes

note

Hickory liquid smoke is available from delicatessens and speciality grocery stores.

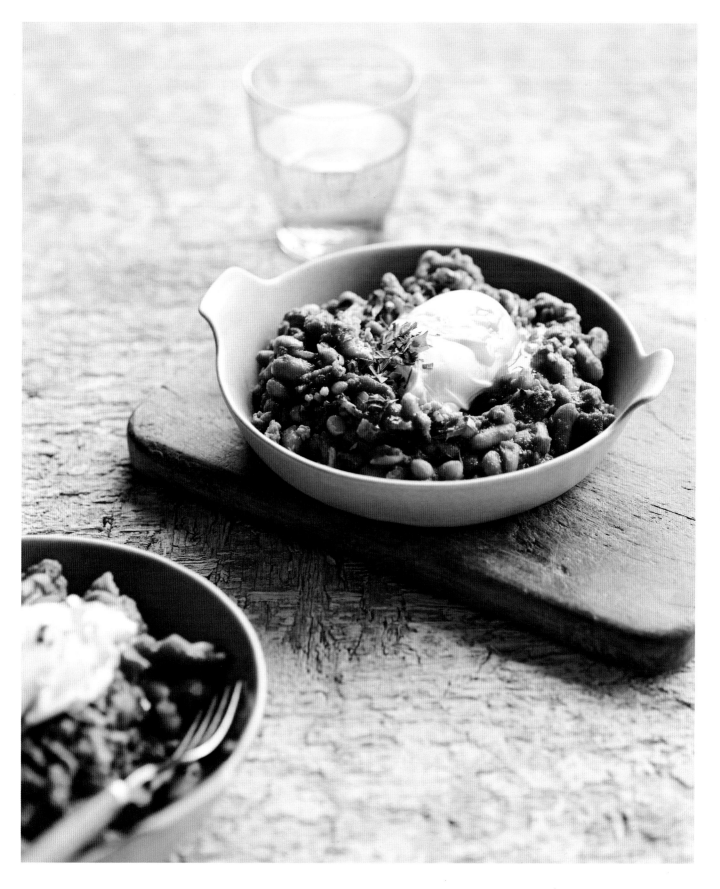

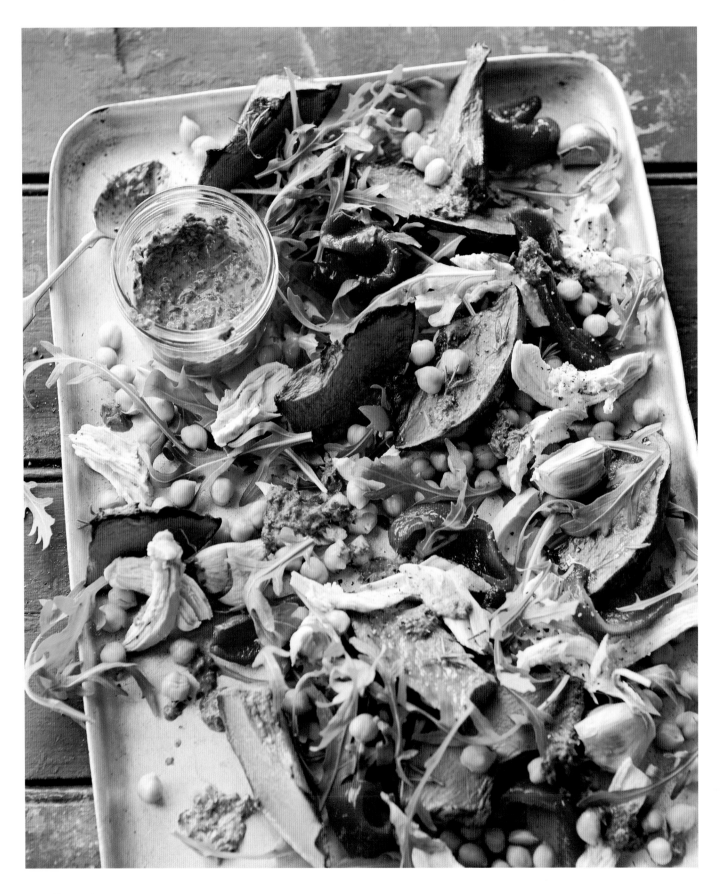

POACHED CHICKEN *with* ROASTED PUMPKIN *and* HERB DRESSING

The chickpeas make this dish moderate in low-GI carbohydrate and high in fibre and potassium.

Ingredients

700 g (1 lb 9 oz) jap or kent pumpkin (winter squash), unpeeled, thickly sliced

8 garlic cloves, unpeeled

2 tablespoons chopped rosemary leaves

3 large red capsicums (peppers), halved

4 x 125 g (4½ oz) skinless chicken breast fillets

1 small brown onion, chopped

1 celery stalk, chopped

1 carrot, chopped

4 thyme sprigs

80 g (2¾ oz) baby rocket (arugula)

400 g (14 oz) tinned no-added-salt chickpeas, rinsed and drained

Herb dressing

1 large handful parsley leaves

1 large handful basil leaves

1 small handful oregano leaves

1 small handful mint leaves

60 ml (2 fl oz/¼ cup) lemon juice

2 anchovies in oil, drained

1 tablespoon extra virgin olive oil

Method

1 Preheat the oven to 200°C (400°F). Line two baking trays with baking paper. Arrange the pumpkin and garlic on one tray, season with freshly ground black pepper and sprinkle with the rosemary. Arrange the capsicums, cut side down, on the other tray. Put the capsicums on the highest oven shelf and the pumpkin underneath. Bake for 30–35 minutes or until the pumpkin is tender and the capsicums start to blacken.

2 Wrap the capsicums in foil and set aside to sweat for 10 minutes. When cool enough to handle, peel away the skins and thickly slice the flesh.

3 Put the chicken, onion, celery, carrot, thyme and 750 ml (26 fl oz/3 cups) water in a saucepan over low heat. Cover and simmer for 15 minutes or until the chicken is cooked through. Leave the chicken in the liquid for 10 minutes before transferring to a plate. Using clean hands, shred the chicken.

4 To make the herb dressing, use a food processor or stick blender to blend the herbs, lemon juice, anchovies and oil until smooth.

5 Arrange the rocket, pumpkin, capsicums, chicken, chickpeas and garlic on a large platter or individual plates. Sprinkle with freshly ground black pepper and drizzle with the herb dressing.

Serves 4

Preparation 20 minutes + cooling

Cooking 50 minutes

Nutrition	Per serve
Energy (kJ)	1995
Protein (g)	42
Carbohydrate (g)	34
Starches (g)	18
Sugars (g)	16
Exchanges	2.5
Portions	3.5
GI	Low
GL	Low
Protein:carbohydrate ratio	1.24
Fat (g)	16
Saturated fat (g)	3
Unsaturated fat (g)	13
Saturated:unsaturated ratio	0.23
Fibre (g)	13
Sodium (mg)	235
Potassium (mg)	1050
Sodium:potassium ratio	0.22
Gluten free?	Yes

notes

Use this poaching method for other recipes needing cooked chicken. The strained poaching liquid makes a tasty stock. Store it in a sealed container in the refrigerator for up to 3 days or in the freezer for up to 3 months. The pumpkin can be substituted with orange sweet potato or parsnips.

FENNEL MEATBALLS *with* ZUCCHINI SPAGHETTI *and* HERB CRUMBS

If you don't have a mandolin, you can prepare the zucchini using a coarse grater. A vegetable peeler can also be used to make zucchini ribbons.

Ingredients

500 g (1 lb 2 oz) lean minced (ground) pork and veal
1 brown onion, finely chopped
2 teaspoons fennel seeds
1 teaspoon chilli flakes
2 garlic cloves, crushed
125 ml (4 fl oz/½ cup) red wine
4 tomatoes, puréed
1 small handful basil leaves, finely chopped
1 small handful parsley leaves, finely chopped
1 small handful oregano leaves, finely chopped
olive oil spray
120 g (4¼ oz) day-old sourdough bread, made into breadcrumbs
4 large zucchini (courgettes), grated or sliced lengthways with a mandolin
2 teaspoons apple cider vinegar
20 g (¾ oz) shaved parmesan cheese

Method

1 Put the pork and veal, onion, fennel seeds, chilli flakes and garlic in a bowl and mix together. Roll tablespoons of the mixture to make 20 balls.

2 Heat a large non-stick frying pan over medium-high heat. Cook the meatballs, turning frequently, for 3–4 minutes or until browned. Pour in the wine and cook for 1 minute or until reduced by half. Stir in the tomato purée, reduce the heat to low and simmer for 30 minutes or until the sauce has thickened. Add half the chopped herbs.

3 Meanwhile, spray another non-stick frying pan with olive oil and place over medium heat. Cook the breadcrumbs, stirring, for 4–5 minutes or until golden and crunchy. Transfer the breadcrumbs to a bowl and stir in the remaining herbs.

4 Spray the frying pan with more olive oil and place over high heat. Cook the zucchini for 2–3 minutes or until just wilted. Stir in the vinegar and season well with freshly ground black pepper.

5 Serve the meatballs and sauce on the zucchini spaghetti, topped with the herbed breadcrumbs and parmesan shavings.

Serves 4
Preparation 40 minutes
Cooking 40 minutes

Nutrition	Per serve
Energy (kJ)	1500
Protein (g)	35
Carbohydrate (g)	23
Starches (g)	14
Sugars (g)	9
Exchanges	1.5
Portions	2.5
GI	Low
GL	Medium
Protein:carbohydrate ratio	1.52
Fat (g)	9.5
Saturated fat (g)	3
Unsaturated fat (g)	6.5
Saturated:unsaturated ratio	0.46
Fibre (g)	9
Sodium (mg)	340
Potassium (mg)	1370
Sodium:potassium ratio	0.25
Gluten free?	No

notes

Add grated carrot and zucchini to the meatballs for an extra serving of vegetables. The meatballs can also be made using lean minced chicken.

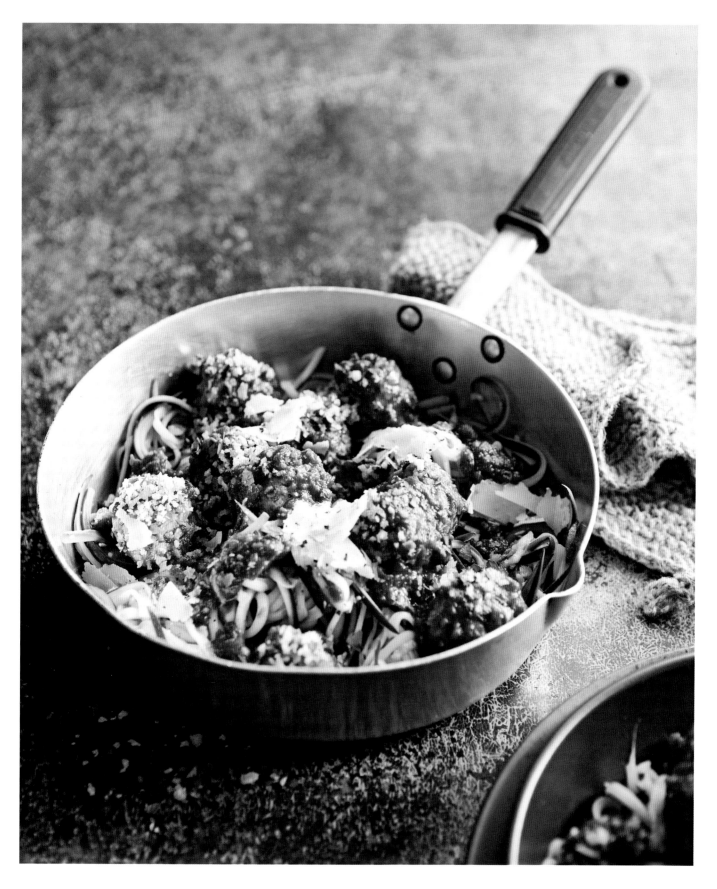

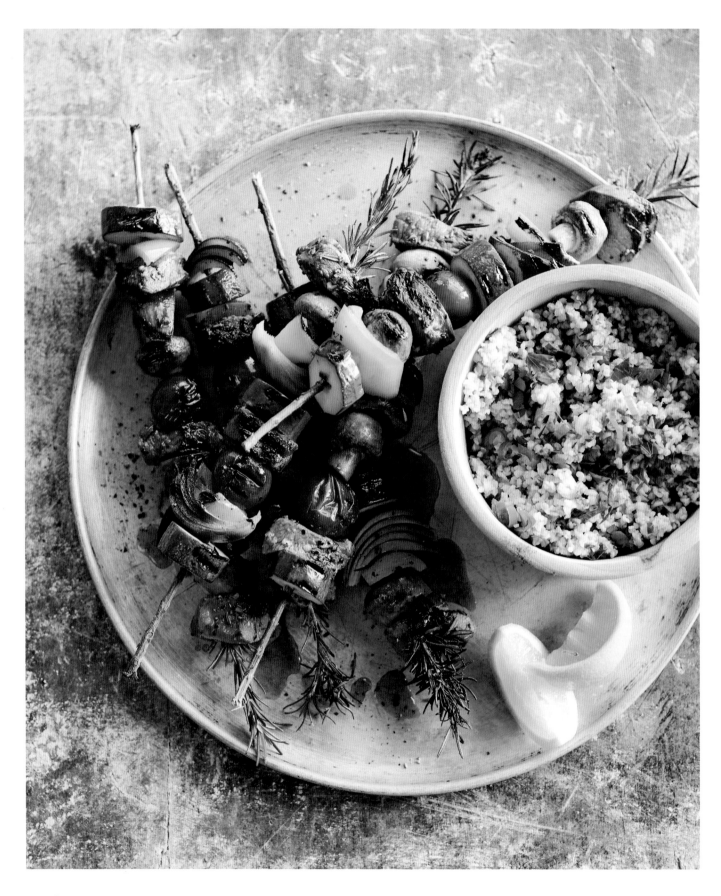

ROSEMARY LAMB *and* VEGETABLE KEBABS *with* LEMON CRACKED WHEAT

This dish is high in protein and moderate in high-fibre, low-GI carbohydrate. It is also a good source of unsaturated fat.

Ingredients

12 rosemary stems
1½ tablespoons olive oil
2 garlic cloves, crushed
2 tablespoons lemon juice
½ teaspoon cracked black pepper
500 g (1 lb 2 oz) lean lamb, cut into 3 cm (1¼ inch) cubes
250 g (9 oz) small button mushrooms
1 large yellow capsicum (pepper), cut into 3 cm (1¼ inch) pieces
1 large red onion, cut into wedges
3 small zucchini (courgettes), thickly sliced
250 g (9 oz) cherry tomatoes
lemon wedges, to serve

Lemon cracked wheat
225 g (8 oz/1 cup) cracked wheat
2 tablespoons lemon juice
2 teaspoons grated lemon zest
2 spring onions (scallions), finely chopped
1 large handful parsley leaves, finely chopped

Method

1 Remove three-quarters of the leaves from the base of each rosemary stem. Finely chop one-third of the leaves, discarding the remaining leaves, and set the stems aside. Place the chopped rosemary, oil, garlic, lemon juice and pepper in a glass bowl and mix to combine. Add the lamb and stir to coat, then cover and refrigerate for 2 hours.

2 Meanwhile, to make the lemon cracked wheat, bring 310 ml (10¾ fl oz/1¼ cups) water to the boil in a saucepan. Add the cracked wheat, reduce the heat and simmer for 15 minutes or until the liquid has been absorbed. Fluff the cracked wheat with a fork, then transfer to a bowl to cool for 15 minutes. Fold in the lemon juice, lemon zest, spring onions and parsley. Cover and refrigerate until needed.

3 Preheat a chargrill pan or barbecue plate to medium. Thread the lamb, mushrooms, capsicum, onion, zucchini and tomatoes onto the rosemary stems. Cook the kebabs, turning occasionally, for 8–10 minutes or until done to your liking.

4 Serve the kebabs with the lemon cracked wheat and lemon wedges.

Serves 4
Preparation 30 minutes +
2 hours marinating and
15 minutes cooling
Cooking 30 minutes

Nutrition	Per serve
Energy (kJ)	2070
Protein (g)	37
Carbohydrate (g)	43
Starches (g)	36
Sugars (g)	7
Exchanges	3
Portions	4.5
GI	Low
GL	Low
Protein:carbohydrate ratio	0.86
Fat (g)	16
Saturated fat (g)	4
Unsaturated fat (g)	12
Saturated:unsaturated ratio	0.33
Fibre (g)	13
Sodium (mg)	100
Potassium (mg)	1280
Sodium:potassium ratio	0.08
Gluten free?	No

notes

If rosemary stems are unavailable, wooden or metal skewers can be used. Soak wooden skewers in water for 30 minutes before use to prevent them from burning during cooking.

BALSAMIC CHICKEN
with POTATO *and* FENNEL BAKE

Fennel is a source of potassium and can be eaten raw or cooked. It has
a slight aniseed flavour, but becomes slightly sweeter when cooked.
The green fronds can also be eaten.

Ingredients

4 x 125 g (4½ oz) skinless
    chicken breast fillets
2 tablespoons balsamic
    vinegar
2 garlic cloves, crushed
olive oil spray
2 large lower-GI potatoes,
    such as Carisma, thinly
    sliced
1 brown onion, thinly sliced
1 large fennel bulb, thinly
    sliced, fronds chopped
60 ml (2 fl oz/¼ cup) dry
    white wine
250 ml (9 fl oz/1 cup)
    reduced-fat evaporated
    milk
finely chopped parsley leaves,
    to serve
400 g (14 oz) asparagus,
    steamed
lemon wedges, to serve

Method

1 Put the chicken in a glass dish with the vinegar
and garlic. Cover and refrigerate for 2 hours.

2 Preheat the oven to 180°C (350°F). Line a baking
tray with baking paper. Lightly spray a 20 cm (8 inch)
square ovenproof dish with olive oil.

3 Combine the potatoes, onion, sliced fennel and
fennel fronds in a large bowl. Pour over the white
wine and evaporated milk, and mix until combined.
Transfer the mixture to the prepared dish. Cover
the dish with a sheet of baking paper followed by
a sheet of foil. Bake for 40 minutes, then remove
the foil and baking paper.

4 Transfer the chicken to the prepared tray, add to
the oven and cook with the uncovered potato bake
for 20 minutes or until the potatoes are tender and
the chicken is browned and cooked through.

5 Slice the chicken and serve with the potato bake,
scattered with chopped parsley and accompanied
by the asparagus and lemon wedges.

Serves 4
Preparation 30 minutes +
2 hours marinating
Cooking 1 hour

Nutrition	Per serve
Energy (kJ)	1500
Protein (g)	38
Carbohydrate (g)	24
Starches (g)	12
Sugars (g)	12
Exchanges	1.5
Portions	2.5
GI	Low
GL	Low
Protein:carbohydrate ratio	1.58
Fat (g)	9
Saturated fat (g)	3
Unsaturated fat (g)	6
Saturated:unsaturated ratio	0.5
Fibre (g)	6
Sodium (mg)	175
Potassium (mg)	1610
Sodium:potassium ratio	0.11
Gluten free?	Yes

notes

*Bring the chicken to room temperature 30 minutes before cooking. You can replace
the potato with orange sweet potato or pumpkin (winter squash). Note that this
will affect the cooking time.*

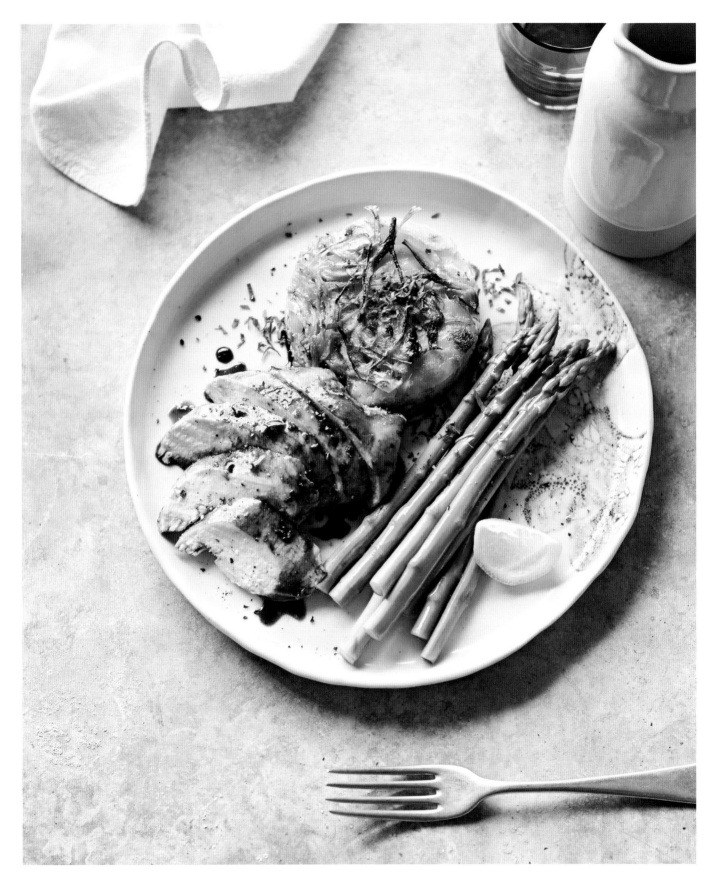

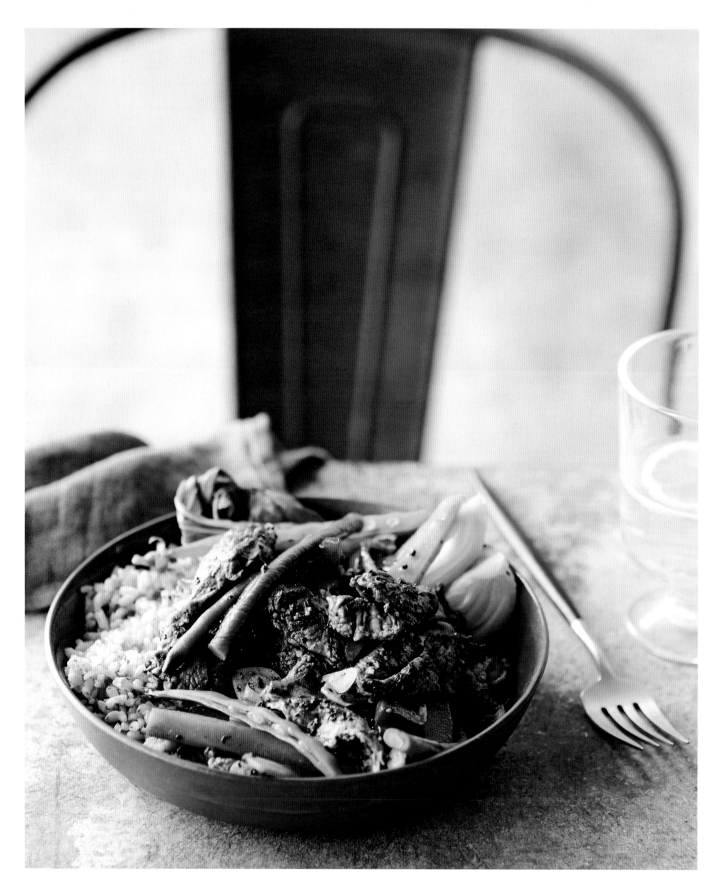

GARLIC, LIME *and* BLACK PEPPER BEEF STIR-FRY

Black pepper has a warm, spicy heat. It is often referred to as the king of spices, having many benefits in addition to improving the overall flavour of many ingredients.

Ingredients

500 g (1 lb 2 oz) lean rump steak, thinly sliced
4 garlic cloves, sliced
2 tablespoons lime juice
2 teaspoons cracked black pepper
canola oil spray
1 carrot, cut into strips
1 red capsicum (pepper), sliced
110 g (3¾ oz) snake (yard-long) beans, cut into short lengths
100 g (3½ oz) snow peas (mangetout), halved
400 g (14 oz) bok choy (pak choy), cut into quarters
370 g (13 oz/2 cups) cooked Doongara low-GI brown rice

Method

1 Put the beef, garlic, lime juice and pepper in a glass bowl. Stir to combine, then set aside to marinate for 15 minutes.

2 Spray a large non-stick wok with canola oil and place over high heat. Stir-fry the marinated beef in two batches for 2–3 minutes or until just cooked. Transfer the beef to a plate.

3 Stir-fry the carrot, capsicum and snake beans in the wok for 5–6 minutes or until slightly softened. Add the snow peas, bok choy and 2 tablespoons water, and stir-fry for 2 minutes or until the greens start to wilt.

4 Return the beef and juices to the wok and cook, stirring, for 1 minute or until well combined and heated through.

5 Serve the beef and vegetables accompanied by the brown rice.

Serves 4
Preparation 15 minutes +
15 minutes marinating
Cooking 15 minutes

Nutrition	Per serve
Energy (kJ)	1500
Protein (g)	34
Carbohydrate (g)	35
Starches (g)	30
Sugars (g)	5
Exchanges	2.5
Portions	3.5
GI	Low
GL	Medium
Protein:carbohydrate ratio	0.97
Fat (g)	8
Saturated fat (g)	3
Unsaturated fat (g)	5
Saturated:unsaturated ratio	0.6
Fibre (g)	6
Sodium (mg)	180
Potassium (mg)	1050
Sodium:potassium ratio	0.17
Gluten free?	Yes

notes

Chicken or pork fillet can be used instead of the beef. Try adding Thai basil, lemongrass or coriander (cilantro) for extra flavour.

CHICKEN *and* CAULIFLOWER NASI GORENG

Cauliflower 'rice' is made by chopping cauliflower in a food processor until it resembles grains of rice. It's an easy way to boost your vegetable intake, increasing your dietary fibre and potassium intake in the process.

Ingredients

250 g (9 oz) skinless chicken breast fillet, thinly sliced

1 tablespoon kecap manis (sweet soy sauce)

1 small (1 kg/2 lb 4 oz) cauliflower, roughly chopped

1½ tablespoons peanut oil

4 raw prawns (shrimp), peeled and deveined, tails intact

2 eggs, lightly whisked

1 red onion, sliced

2 garlic cloves, chopped

½ teaspoon shrimp paste

1 tablespoon sambal oelek (chilli paste)

150 g (5½ oz) Chinese cabbage (wong bok), shredded

4 spring onions (scallions), thinly sliced, plus extra to serve

140 g (5 oz/1 cup) frozen peas, thawed

1 tablespoon crisp fried onions or sliced spring onions (scallions)

½ Lebanese (short) cucumber, thinly sliced

lime wedges, to serve

Method

1 Put the chicken in a glass bowl, add 2 teaspoons of the kecap manis and stir to combine. Cover and refrigerate for 30 minutes.

2 Chop the cauliflower in a food processor in two batches until it resembles coarse rice grains. Don't process the cauliflower too finely or the dish will become too wet. Set aside.

3 Heat 2 teaspoons of the oil in a non-stick wok over high heat. Stir-fry the chicken for 4 minutes or until golden and cooked through. Transfer to a plate. Repeat with another 2 teaspoons of the oil and the prawns. Transfer to a plate.

4 Add 1 teaspoon of the remaining oil to the wok. Pour in the eggs, tilting the wok in a swirling motion to make a thin omelette. Cook for 2 minutes, then carefully turn and cook for a further 2 minutes. Transfer to a plate. When cool enough to handle, roll up the omelette and cut it into thin slices.

5 Heat the remaining 1 teaspoon of oil in the wok over medium–high heat. Stir-fry the onion and garlic for 1 minute. Add the shrimp paste, sambal oelek and remaining 2 teaspoons of kecap manis. Cook, stirring, for 1 minute. Add the cauliflower and stir-fry for 2–3 minutes or until it is starting to soften. Add the cabbage, spring onions and peas, and stir-fry for 3–4 minutes or until the cabbage has wilted. Return the chicken and prawns to the wok and toss to combine.

6 Spoon the nasi goreng into four bowls and serve with the omelette strips, fried onions, extra spring onions, cucumber and lime wedges.

Serves 4

Preparation 20 minutes + 30 minutes marinating

Cooking 25 minutes

Nutrition	Per serve
Energy (kJ)	1400
Protein (g)	31
Carbohydrate (g)	15
Starches (g)	2
Sugars (g)	13
Exchanges	1
Portions	1.5
GI	Low
GL	Low
Protein:carbohydrate ratio	2.1
Fat (g)	15
Saturated fat (g)	3.5
Unsaturated fat (g)	11.5
Saturated:unsaturated ratio	0.3
Fibre (g)	10
Sodium (mg)	500
Potassium (mg)	1340
Sodium:potassium ratio	0.37
Gluten free?	Yes

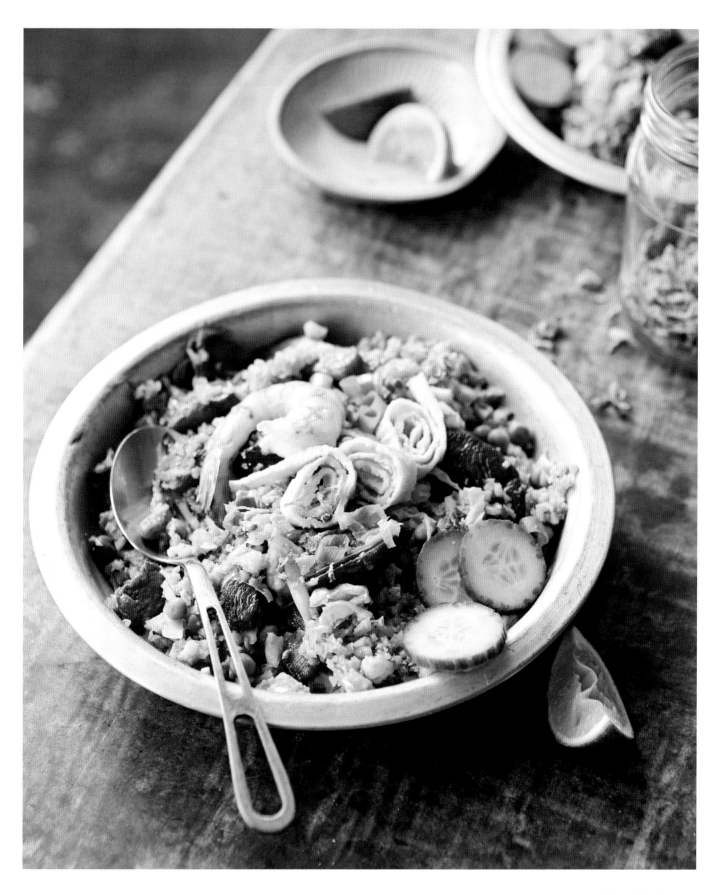

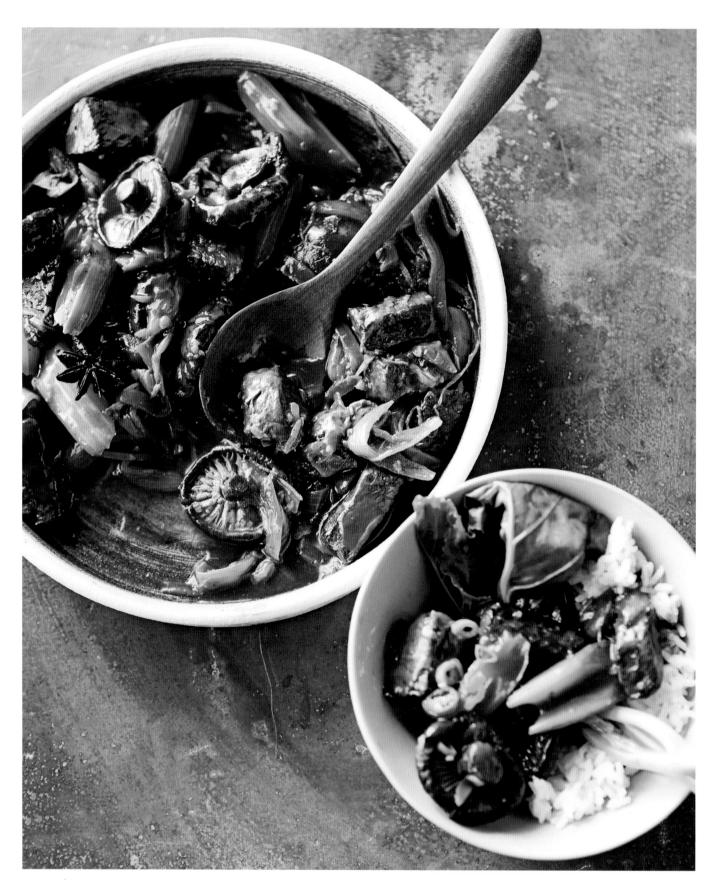

BEEF *and* SHIITAKE MUSHROOMS BRAISED *in* BLACK VINEGAR

Many Asian-style dishes are high in sodium, but this braised beef is not only low in sodium, it's also high in potassium. Black Chinese vinegar (Chinkiang) is made from fermented rice and has a rich, smoky, full flavour.

Ingredients

100 g (3½ oz) dried shiitake mushrooms
olive oil spray
400 g (14 oz) gravy beef, cut into 4 cm (1½ inch) cubes
2 brown onions, sliced
4 celery stalks, thickly sliced
4 garlic cloves, crushed
40 g (1½ oz) piece fresh ginger, grated
2 star anise
1 cinnamon stick
60 ml (2 fl oz/¼ cup) black Chinese vinegar
125 ml (4 fl oz/½ cup) Chinese rice wine
4 spring onions (scallions), thinly sliced
1 long red chilli, thinly sliced
185 g (6½ oz/1 cup) cooked Doongara low-GI white rice
400 g (14 oz) Asian greens, steamed

Method

1 Rinse the mushrooms and put in a heatproof bowl. Cover with plenty of boiling water and set aside for 1 hour to rehydrate. Drain the mushrooms, reserving 250 ml (9 fl oz/1 cup) of the soaking liquid.

2 Preheat the oven to 160°C (315°F). Spray a large flameproof casserole dish with olive oil and place over high heat. Brown the beef in two batches, then transfer to a plate.

3 Add the onions, celery, garlic, ginger, star anise and cinnamon stick to the casserole dish. Cook, stirring, for 4 minutes or until tender and aromatic. Stir in the Chinese vinegar, rice wine and reserved soaking liquid. Return the beef to the dish and add the mushrooms. Cover and transfer to the oven for 2 hours or until the beef is tender and falling apart. Check the beef after 1½ hours and add about 125 ml (4 fl oz/½ cup) water if it is becoming too dry.

4 Serve the beef and mushrooms topped with the spring onions and chilli, accompanied by the rice and steamed Asian greens.

Serves 4
Preparation 15 minutes +
1 hour soaking
Cooking 2¼ hours

Nutrition	Per serve
Energy (kJ)	1455
Protein (g)	32
Carbohydrate (g)	36
Starches (g)	31
Sugars (g)	5
Exchanges	2.5
Portions	3.5
GI	Low
GL	Low
Protein:carbohydrate ratio	0.89
Fat (g)	6
Saturated fat (g)	1.5
Unsaturated fat (g)	4.5
Saturated:unsaturated ratio	0.33
Fibre (g)	7
Sodium (mg)	225
Potassium (mg)	1000
Sodium:potassium ratio	0.23
Gluten free?	Yes

note

Black Chinese vinegar can be bought in the Asian aisle of most supermarkets and from Asian grocery stores and gourmet delicatessens. Balsamic vinegar can be used as a substitute.

LAMB SEEKH KEBABS
with MINTED YOGHURT

Substitute the lamb with lean chicken, pork or beef. If you prefer less heat, omit the chillies from the kebabs and the minted yoghurt.

Ingredients

1 small brown onion, chopped
2 garlic cloves, chopped
30 g (1 oz) piece fresh ginger, grated
2 teaspoons ground cumin
1 teaspoon ground coriander
1 teaspoon garam masala
1 teaspoon red Kashmiri chilli powder
2 long green chillies, seeded and chopped
350 g (12 oz) extra lean minced (ground) lamb
1 egg
2 tablespoons chickpea flour (besan)
250 g (9 oz) cabbage, shredded
1 small red onion, sliced into rings
1 handful coriander (cilantro) leaves
1 lemon, cut into wedges
4 wholemeal (whole-wheat) pitta bread pockets

Minted yoghurt

250 g (9 oz) low-fat plain yoghurt
1 handful mint leaves, chopped
1 handful coriander (cilantro) leaves, chopped
1 small green chilli, seeded and finely chopped

Method

1 Combine the chopped onion, garlic, ginger, spices and green chillies in the bowl of a food processor. Chop until a paste is formed. Add the lamb, egg and chickpea flour, and chop until just combined. Season the mixture with freshly ground black pepper.

2 Divide the lamb mixture into four portions. Using damp hands, roll each portion into a 15 cm (6 inch) log. Thread each log onto a metal skewer. Cover with plastic wrap and refrigerate for 1 hour.

3 Meanwhile, to make the minted yoghurt, mix the yoghurt, mint, coriander and chilli in a small bowl. Cover and refrigerate until needed.

4 Preheat a barbecue or chargrill pan to medium–high. Cook the lamb kebabs, turning frequently, for 12–15 minutes or until they are golden brown and cooked through.

5 To serve, slide the kebabs off the skewers. Arrange on a platter with the minted yoghurt, cabbage, onion rings, coriander, lemon wedges and pitta bread.

Serves 4
Preparation 20 minutes +
1 hour chilling
Cooking 15 minutes

Nutrition	Per serve
Energy (kJ)	1745
Protein (g)	32
Carbohydrate (g)	43
Starches (g)	32
Sugars (g)	11
Exchanges	3
Portions	4.5
GI	Low
GL	Medium
Protein:carbohydrate ratio	0.74
Fat (g)	10
Saturated fat (g)	3.5
Unsaturated fat (g)	6.5
Saturated:unsaturated ratio	0.54
Fibre (g)	10
Sodium (mg)	480
Potassium (mg)	1110
Sodium:potassium ratio	0.43
Gluten free?	No

notes

Chickpea flour is made from ground chickpeas and can be found in Asian grocery stores or health food stores. You can substitute the Kashmiri chilli powder with 1 teaspoon of mild chilli powder.

BAKED LEMON THYME CHICKEN
with SUMAC PUMPKIN *and* SPINACH

Sumac comes from the berries of wild bushes native to the Middle East and the Mediterranean. It has a vibrant colour with a fresh lemony zing. This relatively high protein dish is a good source of dietary fibre and potassium.

Ingredients

4 x 125 g (4½ oz) boneless, skinless chicken thigh fillets

60 ml (2 fl oz/¼ cup) lemon juice

2 tablespoons dry sherry

4 lemon thyme sprigs, plus extra to serve

1 lemon, sliced

500 g (1 lb 2 oz) butternut pumpkin (squash), cut into 3 cm (1¼ inch) pieces

olive oil spray

2 teaspoons sumac

700 g (1 lb 9 oz/2 bunches) English spinach

1 tablespoon reduced-fat cooking cream

¼ teaspoon freshly grated nutmeg

Method

1 Preheat the oven to 180°C (350°F). Line a baking tray with baking paper. Put the chicken in a single layer in a small ovenproof dish. Pour over the lemon juice and sherry, then top the chicken with the lemon thyme sprigs and lemon slices.

2 Arrange the pumpkin on the prepared tray. Spray with olive oil and sprinkle with the sumac and some freshly ground black pepper.

3 Bake the chicken and pumpkin for 30 minutes, swapping the trays over halfway, or until golden and cooked through.

4 When the chicken and pumpkin are almost ready, chop the spinach leaves in half and rinse with water. Heat a saucepan over high heat. Add the spinach with the water clinging to the leaves and cook for 1–2 minutes or until wilted. Stir in the cream and grated nutmeg.

5 Arrange the chicken, pumpkin and spinach on four serving plates. Drizzle the chicken with the cooking juices and scatter over the extra lemon thyme to serve.

Serves 4
Preparation 20 minutes
Cooking 30 minutes

Nutrition	Per serve
Energy (kJ)	1220
Protein (g)	30
Carbohydrate (g)	9
Starches (g)	1
Sugars (g)	8
Exchanges	0.5
Portions	1
GI	Low
GL	Low
Protein:carbohydrate ratio	3.33
Fat (g)	12
Saturated fat (g)	4
Unsaturated fat (g)	8
Saturated:unsaturated ratio	0.5
Fibre (g)	6
Sodium (mg)	155
Potassium (mg)	1450
Sodium:potassium ratio	0.11
Gluten free?	Yes

SPICED VEGETABLE PILAF *with* LAMB FILLETS

The dried spices give this pilaf lots of flavour. Toasting the spices helps release their natural aromatics.

Ingredients

1 tablespoon canola oil

2 large red onions, thinly sliced

40 g (1½ oz) piece fresh ginger, finely shredded

2 teaspoons cumin seeds

1 teaspoon ground coriander

1 teaspoon mild chilli powder

½ teaspoon ground cardamom

½ teaspoon freshly ground black pepper

¼ teaspoon ground cloves

¼ teaspoon ground cinnamon

200 g (7 oz/1 cup) Doongara low-GI brown rice

olive oil spray

2 x 200 g (7 oz) lamb backstraps or loin fillet

2 carrots, cut into thin strips

200 g (7 oz) green beans, halved

80 g (2¾ oz/1¾ cups) baby English spinach leaves

1 handful coriander (cilantro) leaves, plus extra to serve

2 tablespoons flaked almonds, toasted

120 g (4¼ oz) reduced-fat plain yoghurt

lemon wedges, to serve

Method

1 Heat the canola oil in a saucepan over medium–high heat. Cook the onions, stirring, for 2–3 minutes or until softened. Add the ginger and spices, and stir for 2 minutes or until browned and aromatic. Stir in the rice and 375 ml (13 fl oz/1½ cups) water, then reduce the heat to low, cover and simmer for 12–15 minutes or until the water has been absorbed. Fluff the rice with a fork, then cover and set aside for 10 minutes.

2 Spray a large frying pan with olive oil and place over medium–high heat. Cook the lamb backstraps for 2–3 minutes on each side or until browned and done to your liking. Transfer to a plate and cover with foil.

3 Add the carrots and beans to the frying pan. Cook over medium heat for 2 minutes or until softened. Add the spinach and coriander leaves, and stir for 1 minute or until the spinach has just wilted. Stir the rice through the vegetable mixture until combined.

4 Thickly slice the lamb and arrange on the pilaf. Top with the almonds and extra coriander, and serve with the yoghurt and lemon wedges on the side.

Serves 4
Preparation 20 minutes
Cooking 30 minutes

Nutrition	Per serve
Energy (kJ)	2160
Protein (g)	31
Carbohydrate (g)	52
Starches (g)	42
Sugars (g)	10
Exchanges	3.5
Portions	5
GI	Low
GL	Low
Protein:carbohydrate ratio	0.6
Fat (g)	18
Saturated fat (g)	4
Unsaturated fat (g)	14
Saturated:unsaturated ratio	0.29
Fibre (g)	8.5
Sodium (mg)	165
Potassium (mg)	1000
Sodium:potassium ratio	0.17
Gluten free?	Yes

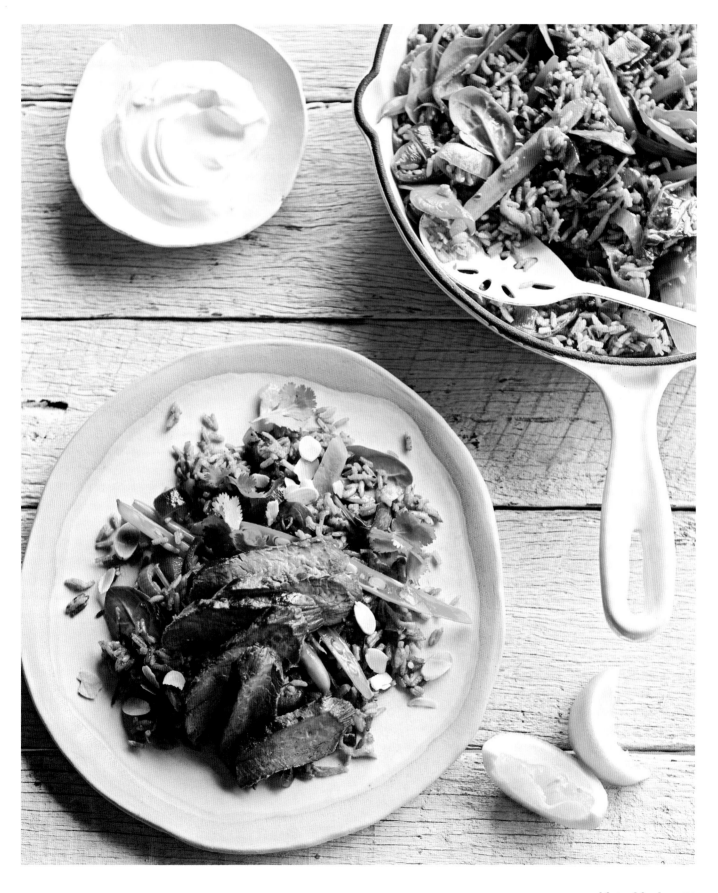

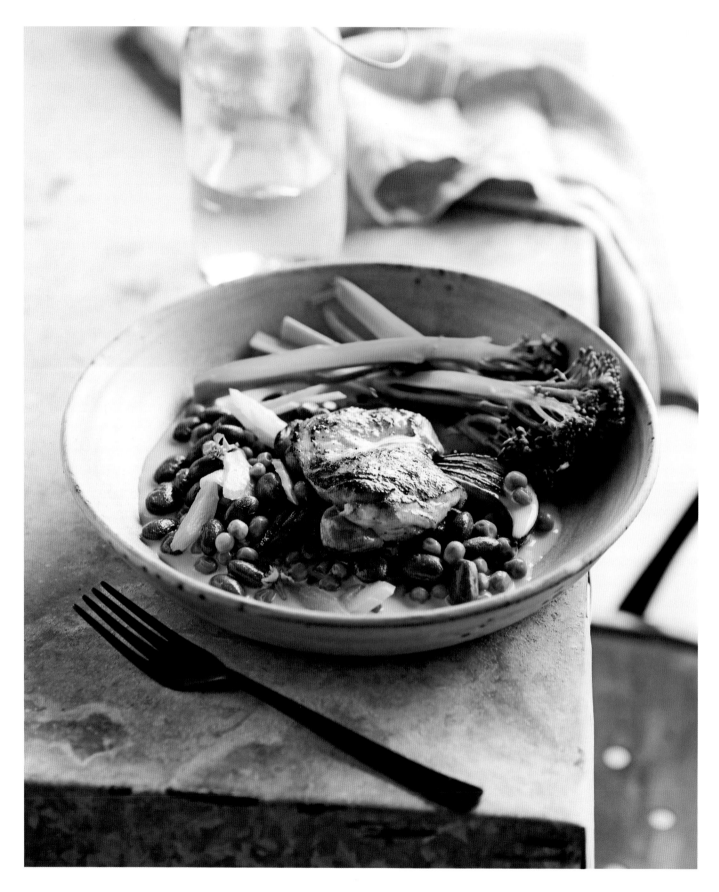

TARRAGON CHICKEN *and* BEANS

Borlotti beans provide a good source of low-GI carbohydrates, B-group vitamins and potassium, and also provide some iron and zinc.

Ingredients

olive oil spray

4 x 120 g (4¼ oz) boneless, skinless chicken thigh fillets, fat trimmed

2 red onions, cut into wedges

2 celery stalks, sliced

125 ml (4 fl oz/½ cup) dry white wine

1 small handful tarragon leaves, plus extra leaves and flowers to serve

800 g (1 lb 12 oz) tinned no-added-salt borlotti beans

125 ml (4 fl oz/½ cup) reduced-fat evaporated milk

140 g (5 oz/1 cup) frozen peas, thawed

400 g (14 oz) broccolini, steamed

Method

1 Spray a large heavy-based saucepan with olive oil and place over medium heat. Cook the chicken for 2 minutes on each side or until browned. Transfer to a plate.

2 Add the onion wedges and celery to the pan and cook, stirring, for 2 minutes or until the onions have softened. Pour in the wine and stir until combined. Return the chicken to the pan, cover and cook for 15 minutes or until the chicken is cooked through.

3 Add the tarragon leaves, borlotti beans, evaporated milk and peas to the pan and cook for 10 minutes or until the sauce is thickened and heated through.

4 Sprinkle the chicken and beans with the extra tarragon and serve with the broccolini.

Serves 4
Preparation 15 minutes
Cooking 35 minutes

Nutrition	Per serve
Energy (kJ)	2465
Protein (g)	50
Carbohydrate (g)	63
Starches (g)	53
Sugars (g)	10
Exchanges	4
Portions	6.5
GI	Low
GL	Medium
Protein:carbohydrate ratio	0.79
Fat (g)	12
Saturated fat (g)	4
Unsaturated fat (g)	8
Saturated:unsaturated ratio	0.5
Fibre (g)	14
Sodium (mg)	200
Potassium (mg)	1800
Sodium:potassium ratio	0.11
Gluten free?	Yes

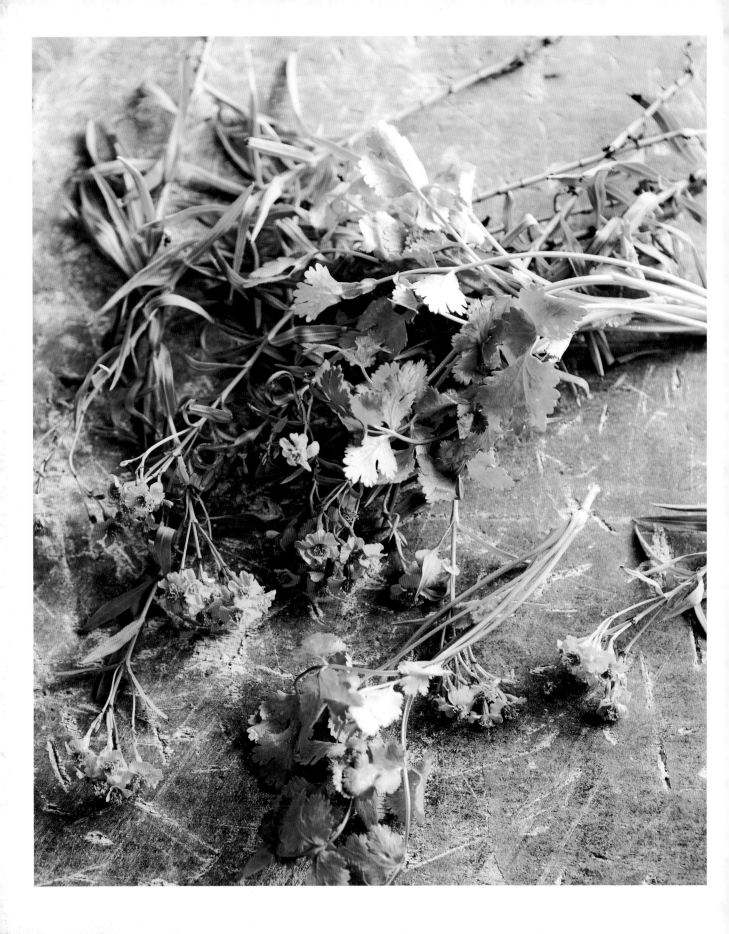

Chapter Six
EASY ENTERTAINING

STUFFED EGGPLANTS

Relatively low in kilojoules, fat and sodium, and high in potassium, this is an ideal appetiser for a special meal. For a vegetarian option, omit the meat and add vegetables such as peas, grated carrots and orange sweet potato.

Ingredients

100 g (3½ oz/½ cup) red lentils
3 x 350 g (12 oz) eggplants (aubergines)
olive oil spray
1 brown onion, finely chopped
250 g (9 oz) lean minced (ground) lamb
300 g (10½ oz) cherry tomatoes, chopped
1 zucchini (courgette), grated
1 tablespoon tomato paste (concentrated purée)
2 tablespoons chopped oregano leaves, plus extra to serve
2 tablespoons chopped mint leaves
1 tablespoon white balsamic vinegar
350 g (12 oz) baby kale leaves

Method

1 Rinse and drain the lentils, discarding any that are discoloured. Transfer them to a small saucepan with 375 ml (13 fl oz/1½ cups) water. Bring to the boil and cook for 10–12 minutes or until the lentils are soft but still holding their shape. Drain and rinse, then set aside until needed.

2 Preheat the oven to 180°C (350°F).

3 Cut the eggplants in half lengthways. Carefully scoop out the flesh with a spoon, leaving a 1 cm (½ inch) shell. Finely chop the eggplant flesh. Put the eggplant halves in a roasting tin, cut side up.

4 Spray a large non-stick frying pan with olive oil and place over medium heat. Cook the chopped eggplant for 6–7 minutes or until it is tender and browned. Transfer to a plate. Add the chopped onion to the pan and cook, stirring, for 2 minutes or until softened. Add the lamb and cook, stirring and breaking up lumps, for 3–4 minutes or until browned. Stir in the tomatoes, zucchini, tomato paste and 80 ml (2½ fl oz/⅓ cup) water, and cook for 2–3 minutes or until all the vegetables have softened. Stir in the lentils, eggplant, oregano, mint and balsamic vinegar until well combined.

5 Fill the eggplant halves with the lamb mixture. Pour 250 ml (9 fl oz/1 cup) water into the base of the roasting tin and bake the eggplants for 1 hour or until tender.

6 Sprinkle the eggplants with the extra oregano and serve with the baby kale leaves.

Serves 6
Preparation 30 minutes
Cooking 1½ hours

Nutrition	Per serve
Energy (kJ)	770
Protein (g)	16
Carbohydrate (g)	15
Starches (g)	6
Sugars (g)	9
Exchanges	1
Portions	1.5
GI	Low
GL	Low
Protein:carbohydrate ratio	1.1
Fat (g)	4.5
Saturated fat (g)	1.5
Unsaturated fat (g)	3
Saturated:unsaturated ratio	0.5
Fibre (g)	10.5
Sodium (mg)	80
Potassium (mg)	975
Sodium:potassium ratio	0.08
Gluten free?	Yes

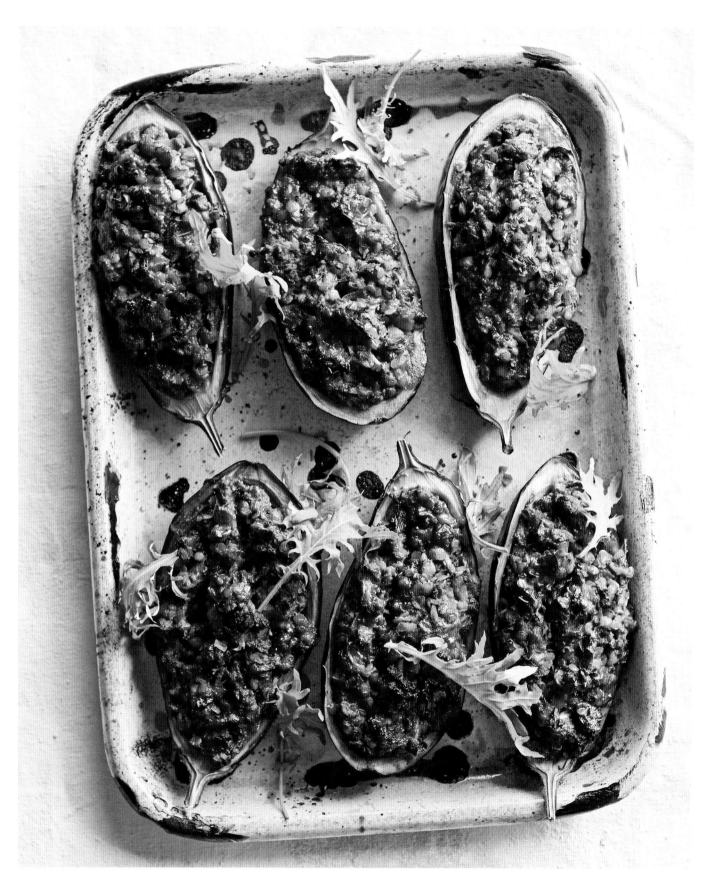

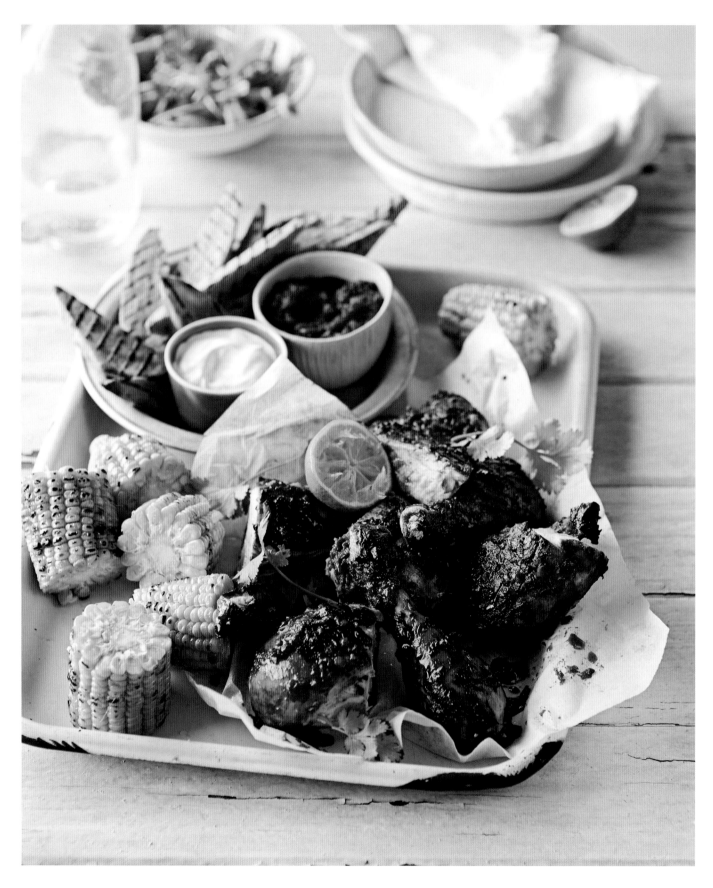

CHIPOTLE BARBECUED CHICKEN
with SWEET POTATO WEDGES

Chipotle chillies in adobo sauce are dried, smoked red jalapeños in a spicy tomato sauce. You can find these in tins in speciality grocery stores and gourmet delicatessens.

Ingredients

2 tablespoons chipotle chillies in adobo sauce

2 ripe tomatoes, chopped

1 red onion, roughly chopped

60 ml (2 fl oz/¼ cup) apple cider vinegar

2 tablespoons yellow box honey

2 tablespoons bourbon

1 tablespoon smoked paprika

2 teaspoons mustard powder

1 handful coriander (cilantro) leaves, plus extra sprigs to serve

1.3 kg (3 lb) whole chicken

500 g (1 lb 2 oz) orange sweet potato, cut into wedges

olive oil spray

2 corn cobs, cut into thirds

125 g (4½ oz/½ cup) extra light sour cream

300 g (10½ oz) mixed salad leaves

lime cheeks, to serve

Method

1 Using a stick blender or a small food processor, blend the chillies, tomatoes, onion, vinegar, honey, bourbon, paprika, mustard and coriander leaves to form a thick paste.

2 To butterfly the chicken, use poultry shears to cut down each side of the backbone. Discard the backbone, turn the chicken over and use the palm of your hand to press down on the breastbone to flatten the chicken. Put the chicken in a large glass dish. Rub half of the chilli mixture over the chicken. Cover with plastic wrap and refrigerate overnight. Spoon the remaining chilli mixture into a bowl, cover and refrigerate until required.

3 Preheat a barbecue to low. Remove the chicken from the marinade and dilute the marinade with 2 tablespoons water. Cook the chicken, basting occasionally with the diluted marinade, for 25 minutes on each side or until golden and cooked through. Spray the sweet potato wedges with olive oil and add to the barbecue for the final 25 minutes of cooking, turning occasionally. Spray the corn cob pieces with olive oil and add to the barbecue for the final 10 minutes, turning frequently.

4 Pour the reserved chilli mixture into a saucepan with 60 ml (2 fl oz/¼ cup) water. Cook over medium heat, stirring occasionally, for 3–4 minutes or until thickened. Spoon the sauce into a small bowl.

5 Using a pair of poultry shears, cut the chicken into small portions. Arrange the chicken on a platter and scatter the coriander sprigs over the top. Serve with the sweet potato wedges, corn, sour cream, salad leaves, chilli sauce and lime cheeks.

Serves 6

Preparation 30 minutes + overnight marinating

Cooking 55 minutes

Nutrition	Per serve
Energy (kJ)	2710
Protein (g)	43
Carbohydrate (g)	33
Starches (g)	15
Sugars (g)	17
Exchanges	2
Portions	3.5
GI	Low
GL	Low
Protein:carbohydrate ratio	1.3
Fat (g)	35
Saturated fat (g)	11
Unsaturated fat (g)	24
Saturated:unsaturated ratio	0.46
Fibre (g)	6
Sodium (mg)	265
Potassium (mg)	1445
Sodium:potassium ratio	0.18
Gluten free?	Yes

PULLED PORK *with* BLACK BEAN SALSA *and* FENNEL SLAW

Moderate in low-GI carbohydrate and quality fat, this dish is an excellent source of potassium. The hickory liquid smoke that gives the pork its smoky flavour is available from delicatessens and speciality grocery stores.

Ingredients

2 teaspoons smoked paprika
2 teaspoons dried oregano
1 teaspoon ground fennel
1 teaspoon ground cumin
1 teaspoon chilli flakes
1 teaspoon onion powder
1 teaspoon cracked black
    pepper
500 g (1 lb 2 oz) piece skinless
    lean pork shoulder
olive oil spray
4 large tomatoes, chopped
2 tablespoons apple cider
    vinegar
1 teaspoon hickory liquid
    smoke (optional)
220 g (7¾ oz/1 cup) dried
    black beans, soaked
    overnight
1 avocado, diced
1 small red onion, half diced
    and half thinly sliced
1 jalapeño, finely diced
1 small handful coriander
    (cilantro) leaves, shredded
60 ml (2 fl oz/¼ cup) lime
    juice
1 baby fennel bulb
300 g (10½ oz) savoy cabbage
1 carrot
1 tablespoon reduced-fat
    sour cream
1 tablespoon buttermilk
6 small salt-reduced wholemeal
    (whole-wheat) flatbreads

Method

1 Preheat the oven to 170°C (325°F). Mix the paprika, oregano, fennel, cumin, chilli flakes, onion powder and pepper in a small bowl. Rub the spice mixture into the pork. Spray a flameproof casserole dish with olive oil and place over medium–high heat. Sear the pork for 5 minutes or until browned all over. Stir in the tomatoes, vinegar, liquid smoke (if using) and 185 ml (6 fl oz/¾ cup) water. Cover and cook in the oven for 2½ hours or until the pork is tender and falling apart.

2 Meanwhile, rinse the black beans, add them to a saucepan and pour in enough water to cover them. Bring to the boil, then reduce the heat and simmer for 45 minutes or until the beans are tender. Drain the beans and set aside to cool for 15 minutes. Stir in the avocado, diced onion, jalapeño, coriander leaves and 2 tablespoons of the lime juice. Cover and refrigerate until required.

3 Thinly slice the fennel bulb, keeping the fronds. Shred the cabbage and carrot. Combine the fennel and fronds with the cabbage, carrot and sliced red onion in a large bowl. Mix the sour cream, buttermilk and remaining 1 tablespoon of lime juice together, then season with freshly ground black pepper. Pour over the vegetables and toss to combine.

4 Transfer the pork to a board, cover with foil and rest for 15 minutes. Skim any fat from the surface of the casserole dish. Put the dish over medium heat and cook, stirring occasionally, for 15 minutes or until the sauce has thickened and reduced by a third.

5 Using two forks, coarsely shred the pork. Pour any juices over the pork and serve with the flatbreads, black bean salsa, fennel slaw and sauce.

Serves 6

Preparation 30 minutes +
overnight soaking and
15 minutes resting
Cooking 3 hours

Nutrition	Per serve
Energy (kJ)	2210
Protein (g)	31
Carbohydrate (g)	39
Starches (g)	30
Sugars (g)	9
Exchanges	2.5
Portions	4
GI	Low
GL	Low
Protein:carbohydrate ratio	0.79
Fat (g)	20
Saturated fat (g)	6
Unsaturated fat (g)	14
Saturated:unsaturated ratio	0.43
Fibre (g)	10
Sodium (mg)	325
Potassium (mg)	1360
Sodium:potassium ratio	0.24
Gluten free?	No

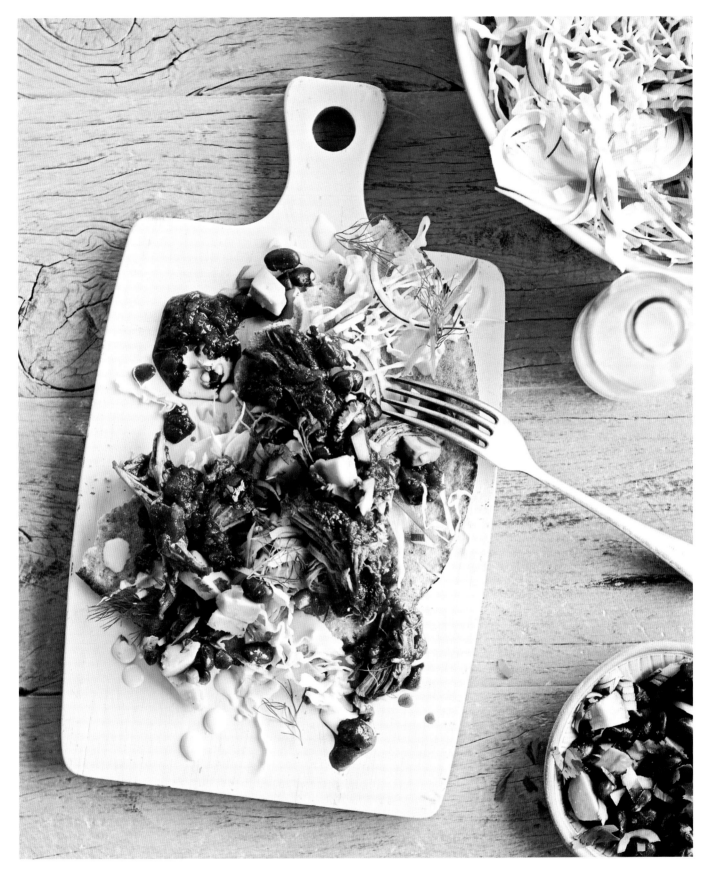

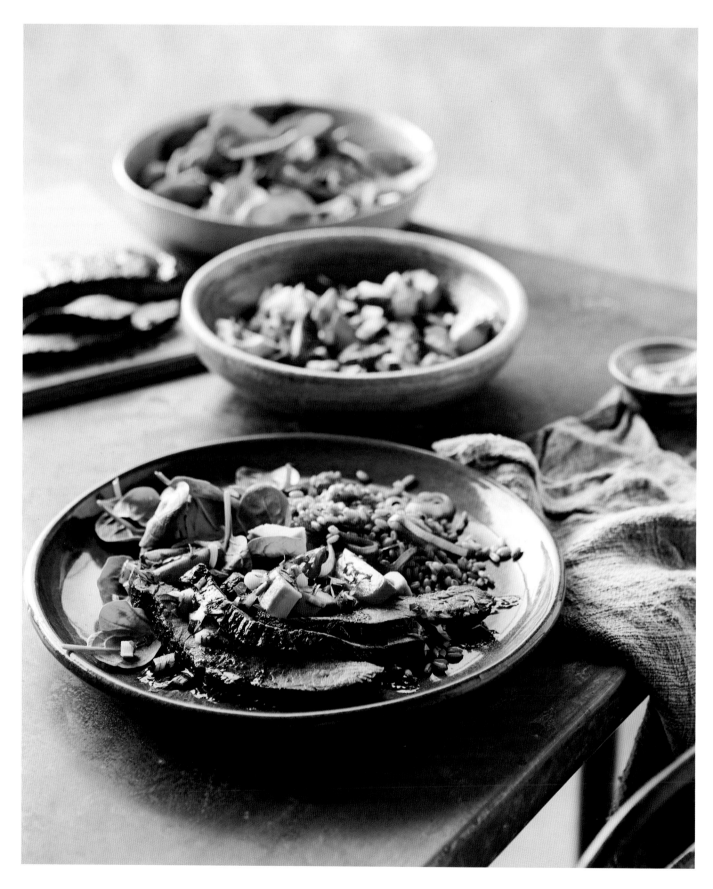

BARBECUED STEAK *with* FARRO *and* TOMATO SALSA

Farro is an ancient, higher-fibre form of wheat. It has a nutty taste and is naturally low in fat.

Ingredients

450 g (1 lb) piece lean skirt steak
2 tablespoons balsamic vinegar
1 tablespoon olive oil
2 teaspoons cracked black pepper
210 g (7½ oz/1 cup) farro
2 French shallots, thinly sliced
60 ml (2 fl oz/¼ cup) red wine vinegar
2 teaspoons hot English mustard powder
80 g (2¾ oz/1¾ cups) baby English spinach leaves

Tomato salsa

250 g (9 oz) baby roma (plum) tomatoes, quartered
½ small red onion, finely diced
1 avocado, finely diced
1 small handful parsley leaves, finely chopped
1 tablespoon lime juice

Method

1 Combine the steak, balsamic vinegar, olive oil and pepper in a shallow glass or ceramic dish. Cover and refrigerate for 1 hour.

2 Combine the farro and 625 ml (21½ fl oz/2½ cups) water in a saucepan. Bring to the boil, then reduce the heat, cover and simmer for 30 minutes or until tender. Drain and rinse under cold water.

3 Put the shallots in a small saucepan with the red wine vinegar and 2 tablespoons water. Cook over high heat for 2 minutes or until the liquid has reduced by a third and the shallots have softened. Set aside to cool, then add the farro and mix until well combined.

4 To make the salsa, combine all the ingredients in a bowl and gently mix together. Set aside.

5 Combine the mustard powder with 2 teaspoons water to form a paste. Set aside.

6 Preheat a barbecue or chargrill pan to high. Cook the beef for 3–4 minutes on each side or until done to your liking. Transfer to a plate, cover with foil and rest for 5 minutes before thinly slicing.

7 Serve the sliced beef topped with the tomato salsa and accompanied by the baby spinach leaves, farro and mustard.

Serves 4

Preparation 25 minutes +
1 hour marinating
Cooking 45 minutes

Nutrition	Per serve
Energy (kJ)	2190
Protein (g)	31
Carbohydrate (g)	35
Starches (g)	32
Sugars (g)	3
Exchanges	2.5
Portions	3.5
GI	Low
GL	Medium
Protein:carbohydrate ratio	0.89
Fat (g)	27
Saturated fat (g)	7
Unsaturated fat (g)	20
Saturated:unsaturated ratio	0.35
Fibre (g)	8
Sodium (mg)	90
Potassium (mg)	1160
Sodium:potassium ratio	0.08
Gluten free?	No

SPICED PEPPER QUAIL
with HERB QUINOA

Quail is a delicate game bird, low in saturated fat and high in protein and iron. It requires minimal cooking time, making it a quick meal to prepare.

Ingredients

200 g (7 oz/1 cup) quinoa, rinsed
2 tablespoons lemon juice
1 tablespoon lemon zest strips
2 tablespoons currants
2 spring onions (scallions), thinly sliced
2 tablespoons flaked almonds, toasted
1 handful parsley leaves, chopped
1 tablespoon plain (all-purpose) flour
¼ teaspoon ground white pepper
¼ teaspoon freshly ground black pepper
¼ teaspoon ground fennel
pinch of Chinese five spice
400 g (14 oz) quail breast fillets, skin removed
olive oil spray
150 g (5½ oz) baby carrots, steamed
250 g (9 oz) broccolini, steamed
lemon wedges, to serve

Method

1 Combine the quinoa and 500 ml (17 fl oz/2 cups) water in a saucepan and put over high heat. Bring to the boil, then reduce the heat to low, cover and simmer for 10–12 minutes or until all the water has evaporated. Transfer the quinoa to a large bowl to cool for 15 minutes.

2 Add the lemon juice, lemon zest, currants, spring onions, almonds and parsley to the quinoa and toss to combine. Set aside.

3 Combine the flour, peppers, fennel and five spice in a plastic bag. Add the quail and shake to coat.

4 Spray a large frying pan with olive oil and heat over medium–high heat. Cook the quail for 2–3 minutes on each side or until golden and cooked through.

5 Serve the quail with the quinoa, carrots, broccolini and lemon wedges.

Serves 4
Preparation 15 minutes +
15 minutes cooling
Cooking 20 minutes

Nutrition	Per serve
Energy (kJ)	1880
Protein (g)	30
Carbohydrate (g)	42
Starches (g)	34
Sugars (g)	8
Exchanges	3
Portions	4
GI	Low
GL	Medium
Protein:carbohydrate ratio	0.71
Fat (g)	16
Saturated fat (g)	3.5
Unsaturated fat (g)	12.5
Saturated:unsaturated ratio	0.28
Fibre (g)	9
Sodium (mg)	85
Potassium (mg)	1200
Sodium:potassium ratio	0.07
Gluten free?	No

notes

Substitute the quail with chicken tenderloins. Instead of serving the quail with steamed vegetables, grated carrots and thinly sliced snow peas (mangetout) can be added to the couscous. Substitute rice flour for a gluten-free version of this dish.

HERB-CRUSTED PORK CUTLETS
with SPICED RED CABBAGE

Add a slightly smoky flavour to this dish by cooking it on a barbecue. You can use any combination of herbs to coat the pork cutlets.

Ingredients

1 small handful parsley leaves, chopped

4 thyme sprigs, chopped, plus extra to serve

4 x 160 g (5½ oz) lean pork cutlets

olive oil spray

60 ml (2 fl oz/¼ cup) freshly squeezed orange juice

400 g (14 oz) tinned no-added-salt cannellini beans, rinsed and drained

80 g (2¾ oz) mixed salad leaves

1 tablespoon lemon juice

Spiced red cabbage

½ small red cabbage, thinly sliced

1 brown onion, thinly sliced

1 green apple, peeled, cored and thinly sliced

30 g (1 oz) piece fresh ginger, grated

¼ teaspoon ground cloves

¼ teaspoon ground cinnamon

¼ teaspoon freshly grated nutmeg

2 tablespoons red wine vinegar

Method

1 To make the spiced red cabbage, heat a large saucepan over medium–low heat. Add the cabbage, onion, apple, ginger, spices, red wine vinegar and 60 ml (2 fl oz/¼ cup) water and gently stir. Cover and cook, stirring occasionally, for 40 minutes or until everything is tender.

2 Use your hands to press the herbs onto the pork cutlets. Spray a non-stick frying pan with olive oil and place over medium heat. Cook the cutlets for 3–4 minutes on each side or until they are golden and cooked through. Remove the cutlets from the pan and cover with foil.

3 Pour the orange juice into the frying pan and boil, stirring for 30 seconds to deglaze the pan. Add the drained cannellini beans and stir for 1 minute or until heated through.

4 Serve the pork on the cannellini beans, drizzled with the pan juices, alongside the spiced cabbage and the salad leaves tossed in the lemon juice.

Serves 4
Preparation 15 minutes
Cooking 50 minutes

Nutrition	Per serve
Energy (kJ)	1415
Protein (g)	46
Carbohydrate (g)	25
Starches (g)	10
Sugars (g)	15
Exchanges	1.5
Portions	2.5
GI	Low
GL	Medium
Protein:carbohydrate ratio	1.84
Fat (g)	3.5
Saturated fat (g)	1
Unsaturated fat (g)	2.5
Saturated:unsaturated ratio	0.4
Fibre (g)	12.5
Sodium (mg)	115
Potassium (mg)	1555
Sodium:potassium ratio	0.07
Gluten free?	Yes

LAMB VINDALOO

This dish is packed full of protein, low-GI carbohydrate and dietary fibre to keep you feeling fuller for longer. Kashmiri chillies are mild in heat. If you like your curry spicy, add a few chopped small fresh red chillies.

Ingredients

400 g (14 oz) diced lamb leg
2 teaspoons ghee
4 ripe tomatoes, finely chopped
2 tablespoons white vinegar
2 tablespoons tamarind purée
2 tablespoons curry leaves
olive oil spray
coriander (cilantro) sprigs, to serve
370 g (13 oz/2 cups) cooked brown basmati rice
Curried cauliflower and green beans with seeds (page 142), to serve

Vindaloo paste

6 dried Kashmiri chillies
5 cm (2 inch) piece cinnamon stick
6 cardamom pods
6 cloves
1 tablespoon cumin seeds
2 teaspoons black peppercorns
1 teaspoon yellow mustard seeds
1 large red onion, roughly chopped
6 garlic cloves, roughly chopped
30 g (1 oz) piece fresh ginger, chopped

Method

1 To make the vindaloo paste, soak the chillies in warm water for 45 minutes. Meanwhile, heat a small heavy-based frying pan over high heat. Dry-fry the whole spices, shaking the pan, for 2 minutes or until aromatic. Cool the mixture for 5 minutes, then blend to a fine powder in a spice mill.

2 Drain and roughly chop the soaked chillies. Put the chillies, onion, garlic, ginger and 2 tablespoons water in the bowl of a food processor and blend to a smooth paste. Combine with the ground spices in a glass bowl.

3 Add the lamb to the vindaloo paste and stir to coat. Cover and refrigerate overnight. Remove from the refrigerator 1 hour before cooking.

4 Heat the ghee in a large heavy-based saucepan over medium–high heat. Remove the lamb from the marinade, reserving the marinade. Cook the lamb, stirring, for 5 minutes or until browned. Stir in the tomatoes, vinegar, tamarind purée, reserved marinade and 125 ml (4 fl oz/½ cup) water. Cover, reduce the heat and simmer, stirring occasionally, for 1 hour or until the lamb is tender. Remove the lid and cook for 30 minutes or until the sauce has thickened and reduced by a third.

5 Heat a small non-stick frying pan over medium–high heat. Spray the curry leaves with olive oil and cook for 1–2 minutes or until crisp.

6 Serve the lamb topped with the curry leaves and coriander, accompanied by the rice and Curried cauliflower and green beans with seeds.

Serves 4

Preparation 40 minutes + 45 minutes soaking and overnight marinating
Cooking 1 hour 40 minutes

Nutrition	Per serve
Energy (kJ)	2745
Protein (g)	47
Carbohydrate (g)	61
Starches (g)	40
Sugars (g)	21
Exchanges	4
Portions	6
GI	Low
GL	Medium
Protein:carbohydrate ratio	0.77
Fat (g)	21
Saturated fat (g)	6
Unsaturated fat (g)	15
Saturated:unsaturated ratio	0.4
Fibre (g)	21
Sodium (mg)	290
Potassium (mg)	1840
Sodium:potassium ratio	0.16
Gluten free?	Yes

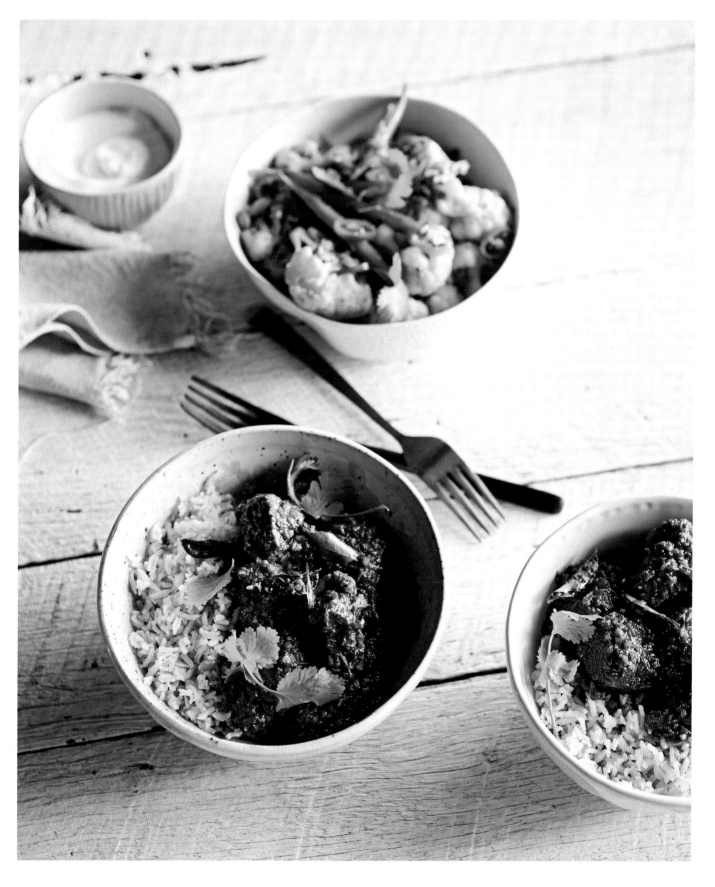

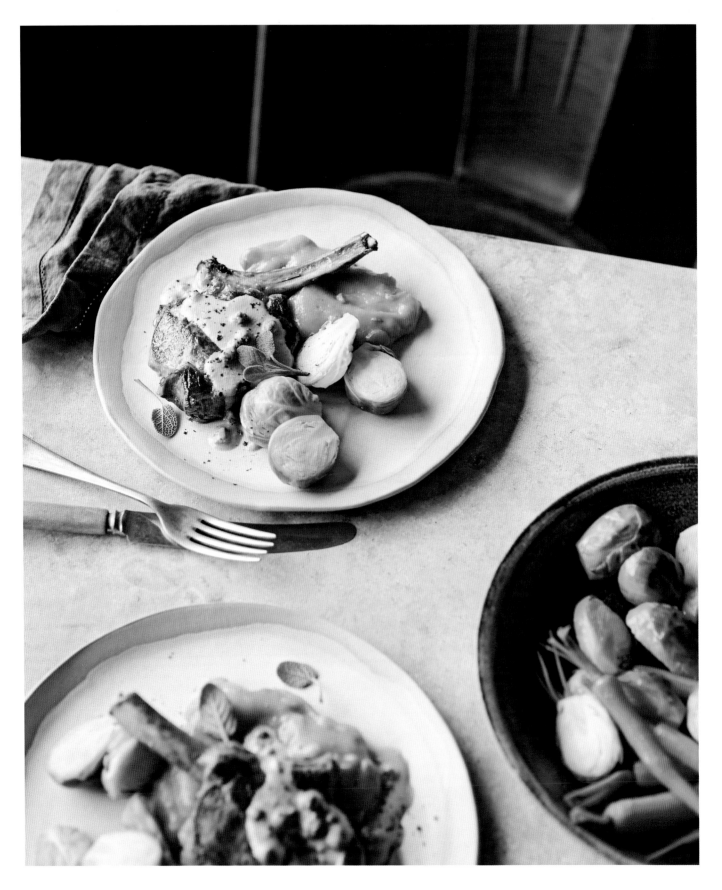

VEAL CUTLETS *with* PUMPKIN *and* SAGE PURÉE

Simple but elegant, this dish makes a lovely winter meal. Lean pork cutlets
can be used instead of the veal cutlets.

Ingredients

500 g (1 lb 2 oz) butternut
  pumpkin (squash), chopped
2 potatoes, chopped
2 spring onions (scallions),
  finely chopped
2 tablespoons skim milk
6 sage leaves, shredded, plus
  extra leaves to serve
olive oil spray
4 x 150 g (5½ oz) lean veal
  cutlets
1 tablespoon baby capers,
  rinsed
1 tablespoon dry Marsala
2 tablespoons reduced-fat
  evaporated milk
300 g (10½ oz) brussels
  sprouts, steamed
400 g (14 oz) baby carrots,
  steamed

Method

1 Cook the chopped pumpkin and potatoes in a
large saucepan of boiling water for 12–15 minutes
or until soft. Drain and use a stick blender to purée
until smooth. Add the spring onions, skim milk and
sage, and stir until well combined and smooth. Cover
and keep warm until serving.

2 Meanwhile, spray a large non-stick frying pan with
olive oil. Place over medium–high heat and cook the
cutlets for 3–4 minutes on each side or until browned
and done to your liking. Transfer to a plate and cover
with foil to keep warm.

3 Add the baby capers, Marsala and evaporated milk
to the pan and cook, stirring, for 1 minute.

4 Spoon the pumpkin purée onto serving plates and
top with the cutlets, sauce and extra sage leaves.
Season with freshly ground black pepper and serve
with the brussels sprouts and carrots.

Serves 4
Preparation 15 minutes
Cooking 20 minutes

Nutrition	Per serve
Energy (kJ)	1540
Protein (g)	43
Carbohydrate (g)	28
Starches (g)	12
Sugars (g)	16
Exchanges	2
Portions	3
GI	Medium
GL	Low
Protein:carbohydrate ratio	1.54
Fat (g)	6
Saturated fat (g)	1.5
Unsaturated fat (g)	4.5
Saturated:unsaturated ratio	0.33
Fibre (g)	10
Sodium (mg)	245
Potassium (mg)	1910
Sodium:potassium ratio	0.13
Gluten free?	Yes

BEEF BOURGUIGNON

Slow cooking tougher cuts of meat over low temperatures gives a very tender end result. Serve the beef with cooked barley as a nutritious alternative to bread.

Ingredients

olive oil spray

600 g (1 lb 5 oz) lean chuck steak, cut into 4 cm (1½ inch) pieces

8 French shallots

1 carrot, thickly sliced

500 g (1 lb 2 oz) button mushrooms, halved

1 lean bacon rasher, thinly sliced

8 garlic cloves

2 tablespoons plain (all-purpose) flour

250 ml (9 fl oz/1 cup) red wine

2 large ripe tomatoes, finely chopped

2 fresh bay leaves

4 thyme sprigs, plus extra to serve

¼ teaspoon freshly ground black pepper

250 ml (9 fl oz/1 cup) boiling water

350 g (12 oz) green beans, steamed

4 thick slices crusty wholegrain bread

Method

1 Spray a large flameproof casserole dish with olive oil and place over medium–high heat. Brown the beef in two batches, then transfer to a plate.

2 Add the shallots to the casserole dish and cook, stirring, for 2–3 minutes, then add the carrot and stir until browned. Transfer the shallots and carrot to a plate. Cook the mushrooms for 4–5 minutes or until browned. Stir in 2 tablespoons water, add the bacon and garlic cloves, and stir for 2 minutes or until golden.

3 Return the beef, shallots, carrot and any juices to the casserole dish, add the flour and stir until combined. Pour in the wine and cook, stirring, for 2 minutes. Add the tomatoes, bay leaves, thyme sprigs, pepper and boiling water. Reduce the heat to low, cover and cook, stirring occasionally, for 1½ hours or until the beef is tender.

4 Serve the beef and vegetables with the extra thyme, steamed green beans and crusty bread.

Serves 4
Preparation 20 minutes
Cooking 1 hour 55 minutes

Nutrition	Per serve
Energy (kJ)	2070
Protein (g)	48
Carbohydrate (g)	25
Starches (g)	20
Sugars (g)	5
Exchanges	1.5
Portions	2.5
GI	Medium
GL	Low
Protein:carbohydrate ratio	1.9
Fat (g)	15
Saturated fat (g)	5
Unsaturated fat (g)	10
Saturated:unsaturated ratio	0.5
Fibre (g)	11
Sodium (mg)	460
Potassium (mg)	1530
Sodium:potassium ratio	0.3
Gluten free?	No

notes

This dish can be prepared a day ahead and refrigerated — the flavour will improve overnight. Reheat it thoroughly before serving. Tie the thyme sprigs together with kitchen string to enable easy removal prior to serving.

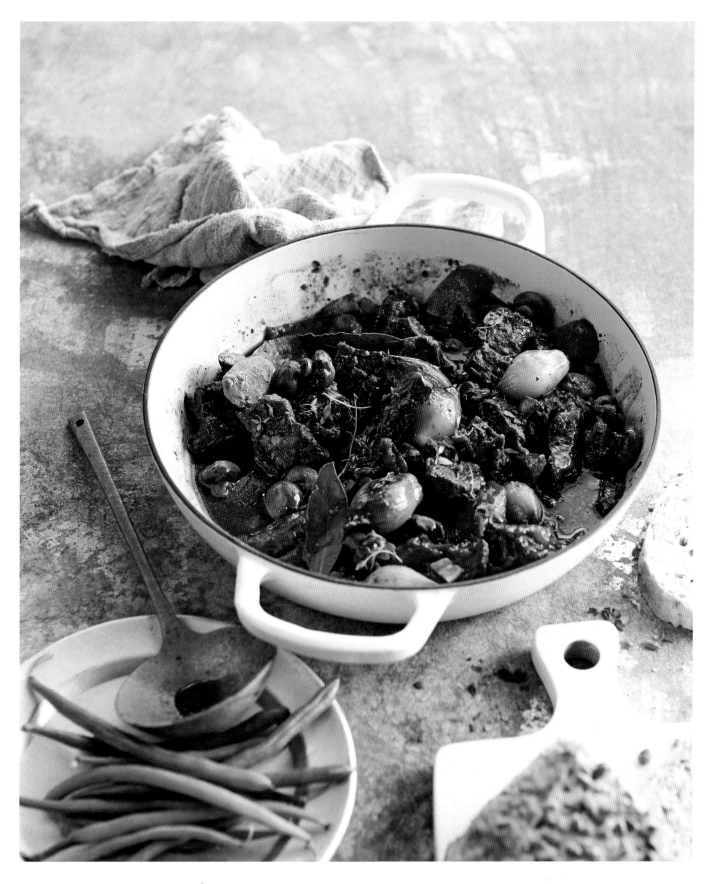

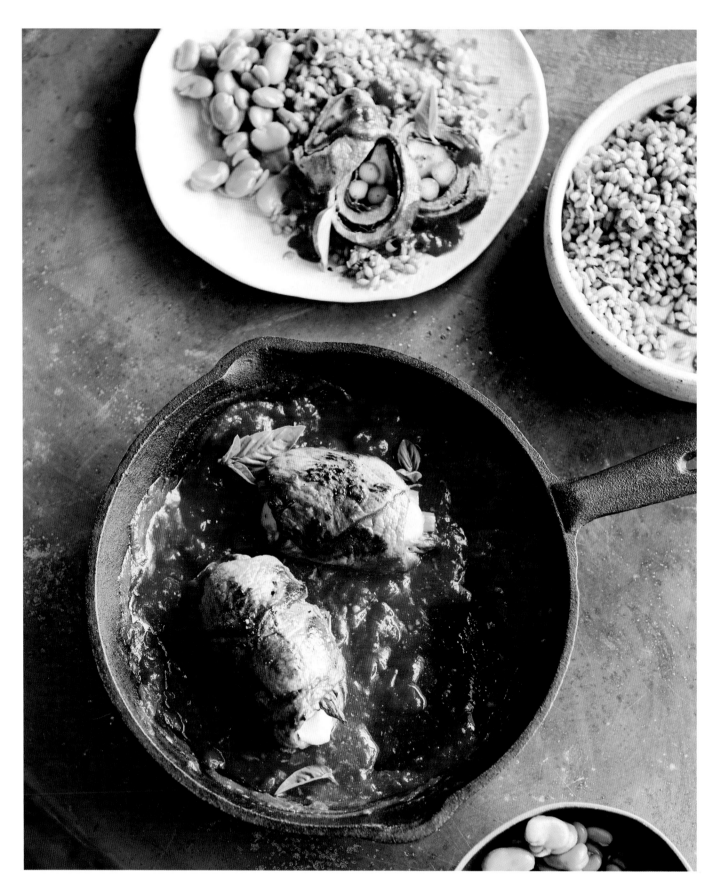

VEAL INVOLTINI *with* BARLEY

These tasty rolls served with herbed barley make a relatively high protein, moderate carbohydrate and high dietary fibre dish that will keep you feeling satisfied for longer.

Ingredients

250 ml (9 fl oz/1 cup) salt-reduced beef stock

125 ml (4 fl oz/½ cup) dry white wine

200 g (7 oz/1 cup) barley, rinsed

2 spring onions (scallions), thinly sliced

1 handful basil, shredded, plus extra leaves to serve

4 x 125 g (4½ oz) veal leg steaks

40 g (1½ oz) baby English spinach leaves

8 (80 g/2¾ oz) bocconcini (fresh baby mozzarella cheese), halved

200 g (7 oz) asparagus spears, trimmed

2 large tomatoes, chopped

1 tablespoon no-added-salt tomato paste (concentrated purée)

olive oil spray

1 tablespoon balsamic vinegar

155 g (5½ oz/1 cup) broad beans, steamed

Method

1 Combine the stock, white wine, barley and 375 ml (13 fl oz/1½ cups) water in a saucepan over high heat. Bring to the boil, stirring, then reduce the heat to low. Simmer, stirring occasionally, for 30–35 minutes or until all the liquid has evaporated and the barley is soft. Stir in the spring onions and shredded basil, cover and set aside.

2 While the barley is cooking, lay the veal steaks on a flat surface and top with the spinach, bocconcini and asparagus. Roll up tightly and secure each roll with a toothpick.

3 Using a stick blender or small food processor, purée the tomatoes and tomato paste until smooth.

4 Spray a non-stick frying pan with olive oil and place over medium heat. Cook the veal, turning frequently, for 3–4 minutes or until browned. Transfer to a plate.

5 Return the frying pan to medium–high heat and add the tomato purée and balsamic vinegar. Cook, stirring occasionally, for 2–3 minutes or until slightly thickened. Return the veal rolls to the pan, cover and cook for 6–8 minutes or until the sauce has thickened and the veal is cooked through.

6 Serve the veal rolls with the barley, tomato sauce and broad beans, topped with extra basil leaves.

Serves 4
Preparation 15 minutes
Cooking 35 minutes

Nutrition	Per serve
Energy (kJ)	1780
Protein (g)	40
Carbohydrate (g)	37
Starches (g)	32
Sugars (g)	5
Exchanges	2.5
Portions	3.5
GI	Low
GL	Low
Protein:carbohydrate ratio	1.08
Fat (g)	8
Saturated fat (g)	3
Unsaturated fat (g)	5
Saturated:unsaturated ratio	0.6
Fibre (g)	10
Sodium (mg)	350
Potassium (mg)	1210
Sodium:potassium ratio	0.29
Gluten free?	No

note

Try using a filling of goat's cheese mixed with chopped walnuts and basil, or use skinless chicken breast fillets sliced horizontally and rolled around a mixture of reduced-fat ricotta cheese, sautéed leek and tarragon.

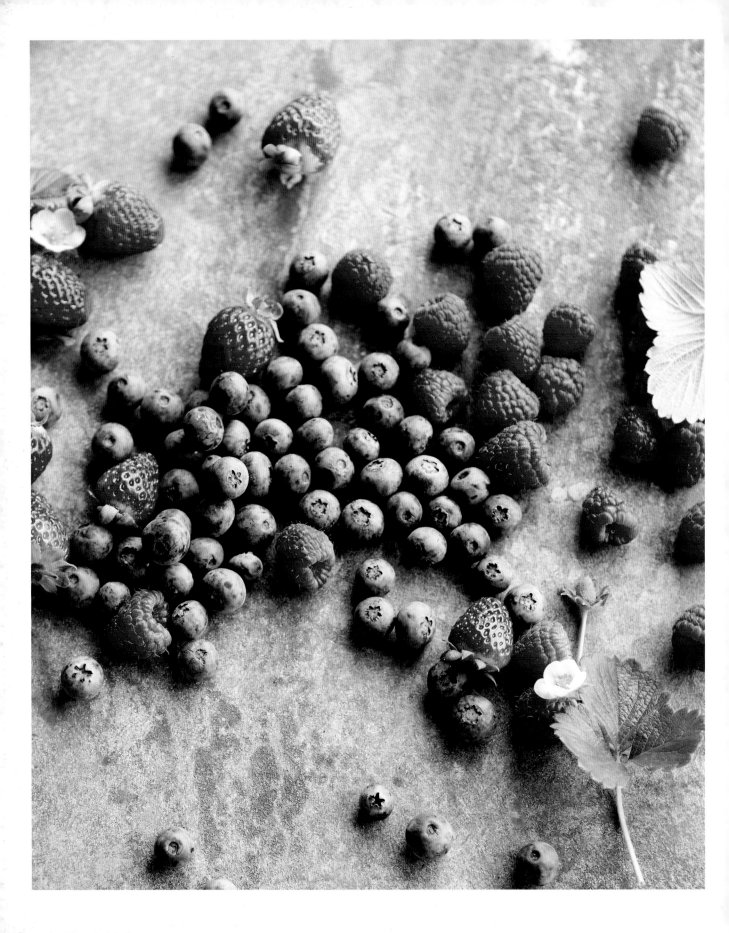

Chapter Seven
SWEET TREATS

CINNAMON OAT BISCUITS

Cinnamon has a long history as a spice and as a medicine. It is loaded with antioxidants and some varieties can help lower blood glucose levels if consumed in large quantities.

Ingredients

100 g (3½ oz/1 cup) rolled (porridge) oats

90 g (3¼ oz/½ cup) spelt flour

35 g (1¼ oz/¼ cup) wholemeal plain (whole-wheat all-purpose) flour

2 tablespoons desiccated coconut

1 tablespoon psyllium husk

1 teaspoon ground cinnamon

50 g (1¾ oz) reduced-fat canola spread

2 tablespoons pure maple syrup

½ teaspoon bicarbonate of soda (baking soda)

1 tablespoon boiling water

Method

1 Preheat the oven to 180°C (350°F). Line a large baking tray with baking paper.

2 Combine the oats, flours, coconut, psyllium husk and cinnamon in a large bowl and make a well in the centre.

3 Heat the canola spread and maple syrup in a small saucepan over low heat until the spread has melted. Set aside to cool for 5 minutes.

4 Dissolve the bicarbonate of soda in the boiling water, then stir into the dry ingredients along with the maple syrup mixture.

5 Roll tablespoons of the mixture to make 12 balls. Put the balls on the baking tray and flatten slightly. Bake the biscuits for 16–18 minutes or until golden and crisp. Transfer to a wire rack to cool before storing in an airtight container for up to a week.

Makes 12
Preparation 15 minutes
Cooking 20 minutes

Nutrition	Per biscuit
Energy (kJ)	450
Protein (g)	3
Carbohydrate (g)	13
Starches (g)	11
Sugars (g)	2
Exchanges	1
Portions	1.5
GI	Low
GL	Low
Protein:carbohydrate ratio	0.23
Fat (g)	4.5
Saturated fat (g)	1.5
Unsaturated fat (g)	3
Saturated:unsaturated ratio	0.5
Fibre (g)	2.5
Sodium (mg)	75
Potassium (mg)	85
Sodium:potassium ratio	0.88
Gluten free?	No

note

Try adding 2 tablespoons unsweetened chopped cranberries or 2 tablespoons chopped almonds.

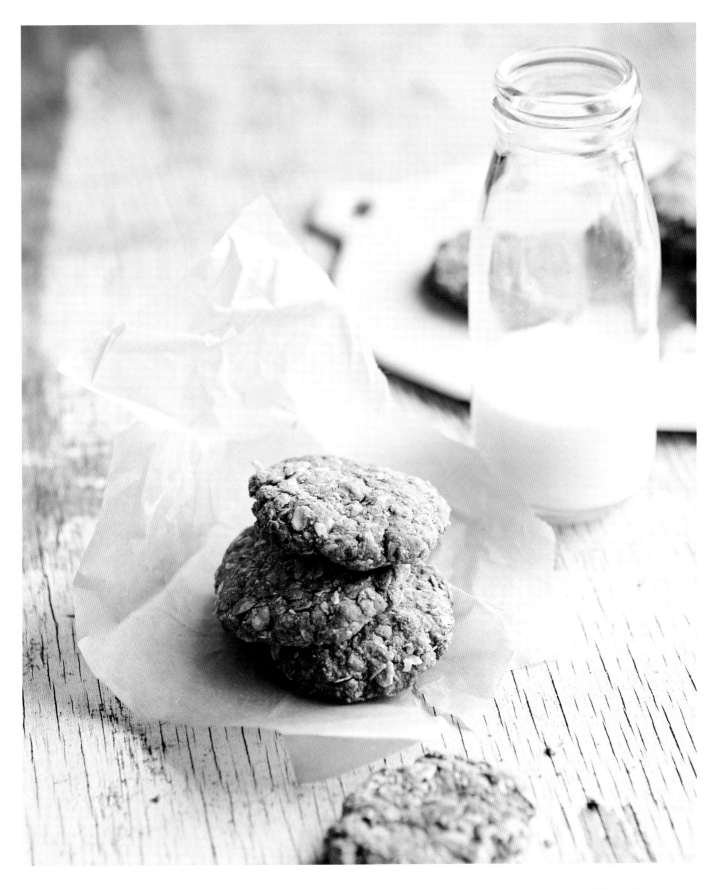

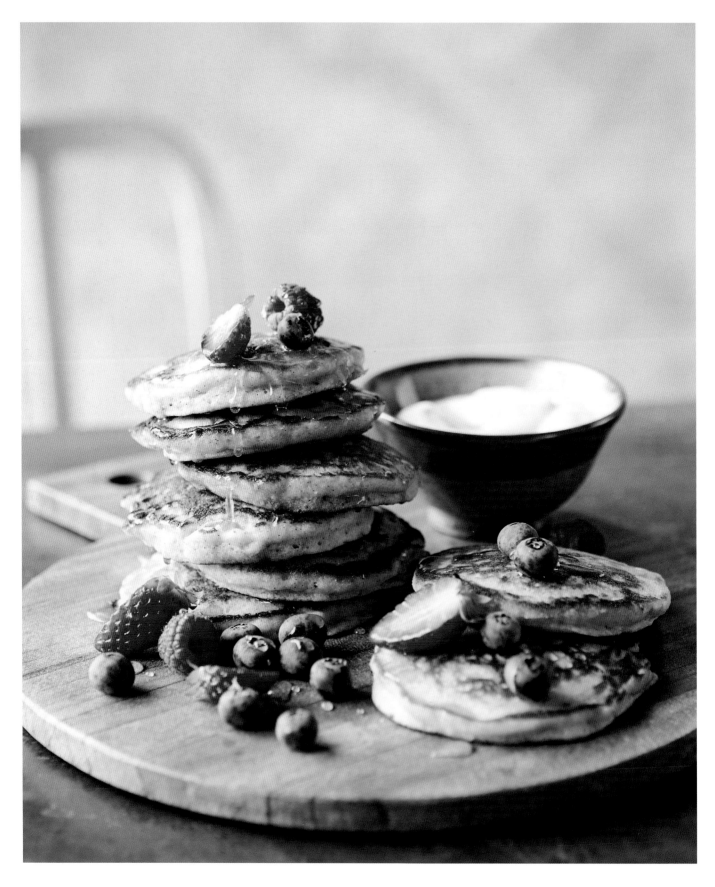

BUCKWHEAT PANCAKES *with* BERRIES

Buckwheat is not related to wheat. It is cultivated from seeds and is therefore a great gluten-free flour. Use gluten-free self-raising flour if you wish to make gluten-free pancakes.

Ingredients

185 ml (6 fl oz/¾ cup) skim milk

1 tablespoon lemon juice

1 tablespoon yellow box honey

1 vanilla bean, split lengthways

100 g (3½ oz/¾ cup) buckwheat flour

35 g (1¼ oz/¼ cup) self-raising flour

2 tablespoons rolled (porridge) oats

2 tablespoons almond meal

½ teaspoon baking powder

2 eggwhites, at room temperature

olive oil spray

200 g (7 oz) mixed fresh berries

130 g (4½ oz/½ cup) low-fat, no-added-sugar vanilla yoghurt

Method

1 Pour the milk into a glass bowl and stir in the lemon juice. Set aside for 10 minutes or until the mixture looks curdled. Add half the honey and the vanilla seeds, and stir until the honey has dissolved.

2 Combine the flours, oats, almond meal and baking powder in a bowl and make a well in the centre.

3 Use an electric mixer with a whisk attachment to whisk the eggwhites in a small bowl until stiff peaks form. Pour the milk mixture into the dry ingredients and mix until just combined. Using a large metal spoon, gently fold in the eggwhites.

4 Spray a large non-stick frying pan with olive oil and place over medium heat. Using 60 ml (2 fl oz/ ¼ cup) of the batter for each pancake, cook the pancakes in batches for 2 minutes on each side or until golden, making eight pancakes in total.

5 Serve the pancakes topped with the remaining honey and the berries, with the yoghurt on the side.

Serves 4
Preparation 15 minutes
Cooking 10 minutes

Nutrition	Per serve
Energy (kJ)	890
Protein (g)	10
Carbohydrate (g)	31
Starches (g)	19
Sugars (g)	12
Exchanges	2
Portions	3
GI	Low
GL	Medium
Protein:carbohydrate ratio	0.32
Fat (g)	4
Saturated fat (g)	0.5
Unsaturated fat (g)	3.5
Saturated:unsaturated ratio	0.14
Fibre (g)	4.5
Sodium (mg)	155
Potassium (mg)	380
Sodium:potassium ratio	0.41
Gluten free?	No

notes

Add a different flavour to the batter by mixing in ¼ teaspoon ground cinnamon and 1 grated apple, or folding in 40 g (1½ oz/¼ cup) blueberries. Vary the topping by crushing frozen raspberries through reduced-fat smooth ricotta cheese.

APPLE CRUMBLES

LSA is a ground mixture of linseeds (flaxseeds), sunflower seeds and almonds. It is a great source of dietary fibre and healthy unsaturated fats, and is sold in health food stores or the health food aisle of supermarkets.

Ingredients

4 small green apples

2 tablespoons frozen mixed berries

35 g (1¼ oz/¼ cup) stone-ground plain (all-purpose) flour

35 g (1¼ oz/¼ cup) LSA

40 g (1½ oz) reduced-fat canola spread

50 g (1¾ oz/½ cup) rolled (porridge) oats

1 teaspoon mixed (pumpkin pie) spice

4 x 1½ tablespoon scoops low-fat, no-added-sugar ice cream, to serve

Method

1 Preheat the oven to 180°C (350°F).

2 Peel, quarter, core and thinly slice the apples. Divide the apples and berries among four 250 ml (9 fl oz/1 cup) capacity ovenproof ramekins.

3 Put the flour and LSA in a small bowl. Using your fingertips, rub in the canola spread until the mixture resembles fine breadcrumbs. Stir in the oats and mixed spice. Sprinkle the mixture over the apples and berries.

4 Bake the crumbles for 25–30 minutes or until the apples are cooked and the tops are golden. Serve warm with the ice cream.

Serves 4
Preparation 30 minutes
Cooking 30 minutes

Nutrition	Per serve
Energy (kJ)	1120
Protein (g)	6
Carbohydrate (g)	28
Starches (g)	14
Sugars (g)	14
Exchanges	2
Portions	3
GI	Low
GL	Medium
Protein:carbohydrate ratio	0.21
Fat (g)	12
Saturated fat (g)	2
Unsaturated fat (g)	10
Saturated:unsaturated ratio	0.2
Fibre (g)	8
Sodium (mg)	60
Potassium (mg)	325
Sodium:potassium ratio	0.18
Gluten free?	No

note

Substitute the berries for sultanas (golden raisins) or unsweetened dried cranberries.

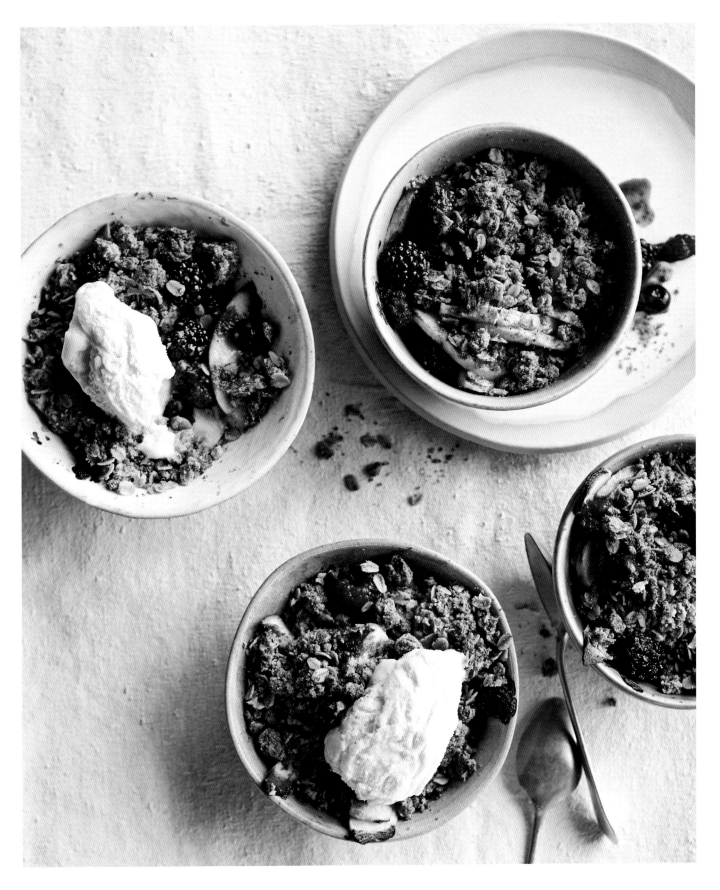

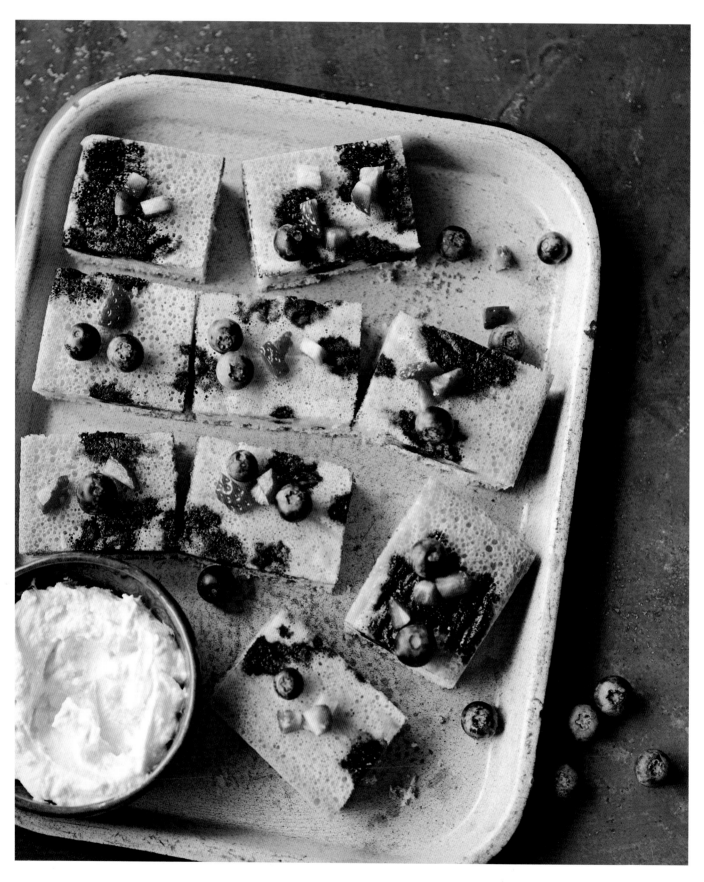

BERRY SPONGE CAKE *with* HONEYED RICOTTA

Blueberries are high in antioxidants and vitamin C. To give the cake a marbled look, purée the frozen berries, then dollop spoonfuls onto the batter and use a metal skewer to swirl the purée through the batter.

Ingredients

canola oil spray

4 eggs, at room temperature

2 tablespoons Splenda sweetener

2 tablespoons self-raising flour

2 tablespoons cornflour (cornstarch)

1 teaspoon cream of tartar

½ teaspoon bicarbonate of soda (baking soda)

25 g (1 oz/¼ cup) almond meal

50 g (1¾ oz/⅓ cup) blueberries

12 strawberries, finely diced

Honeyed ricotta

250 g (9 oz) reduced-fat smooth ricotta cheese

1 tablespoon yellow box honey

1 teaspoon finely grated lemon zest

Method

1 Preheat the oven to 180°C (350°F). Lightly spray a 20 cm (8 inch) square cake tin with canola oil, then line the base and sides with baking paper.

2 Use an electric mixer with a whisk attachment to whisk the eggs and Splenda for 5–6 minutes or until light, fluffy and doubled in size.

3 While the eggs are whisking, combine the flours, cream of tartar and bicarbonate of soda in a bowl. Sift together three times. Stir in the almond meal.

4 Use a large metal spoon to lightly fold the flour mixture through the egg mixture. Pour the batter into the prepared tin and scatter three-quarters of the blueberries on top (they will sink into the batter). Bake for 25 minutes or until the cake is golden and springy to touch. Leave in the tin for 5 minutes, then turn out onto a wire rack. Peel off the paper and leave to cool.

5 To make the honeyed ricotta, beat the ricotta, honey and lemon zest until smooth.

6 Cut the sponge cake into 12 squares and serve topped with the strawberries and the remaining blueberries, with the honeyed ricotta on the side.

Serves 12

Preparation 15 minutes

Cooking 25 minutes

Nutrition	Per serve
Energy (kJ)	385
Protein (g)	6
Carbohydrate (g)	6
Starches (g)	3
Sugars (g)	3
Exchanges	0.5
Portions	0.5
GI	Medium
GL	Low
Protein:carbohydrate ratio	1
Fat (g)	5
Saturated fat (g)	2
Unsaturated fat (g)	3
Saturated:unsaturated ratio	0.67
Fibre (g)	1
Sodium (mg)	135
Potassium (mg)	300
Sodium:potassium ratio	0.45
Gluten free?	No

note

Frozen raspberries or blackberries will also work well in this recipe.

FRENCH APPLE TARTS

These pretty tarts are perfect for a quick and easy dessert. Try using other seasonal fruits, such as peaches, pears or nectarines.

Ingredients

1 large green apple
1 sheet reduced-fat puff
   pastry, just thawed
1 tablespoon hazelnut meal
1 tablespoon yellow box
   honey, warmed
150 g (5½ oz) low-fat,
   no-added-sugar vanilla
   yoghurt

Method

1 Preheat the oven to 200°C (400°F). Line a large baking tray with baking paper.

2 Peel, quarter, core and thinly slice the apple.

3 Using a 10.5 cm (4 inch) round cutter, cut four circles from the pastry. Spread the hazelnut meal over the pastry, then top with the apple slices in a circular pattern. Drizzle the honey over the top.

4 Bake the tarts for 20 minutes or until golden. Serve with the yoghurt.

Serves 4
Preparation 10 minutes
Cooking 20 minutes

Nutrition	Per serve
Energy (kJ)	660
Protein (g)	4
Carbohydrate (g)	24
Starches (g)	11
Sugars (g)	13
Exchanges	1.5
Portions	2.5
GI	Low
GL	Medium
Protein:carbohydrate ratio	0.17
Fat (g)	5
Saturated fat (g)	1.5
Unsaturated fat (g)	3.5
Saturated:unsaturated ratio	0.43
Fibre (g)	2
Sodium (mg)	110
Potassium (mg)	200
Sodium:potassium ratio	0.55
Gluten free?	No

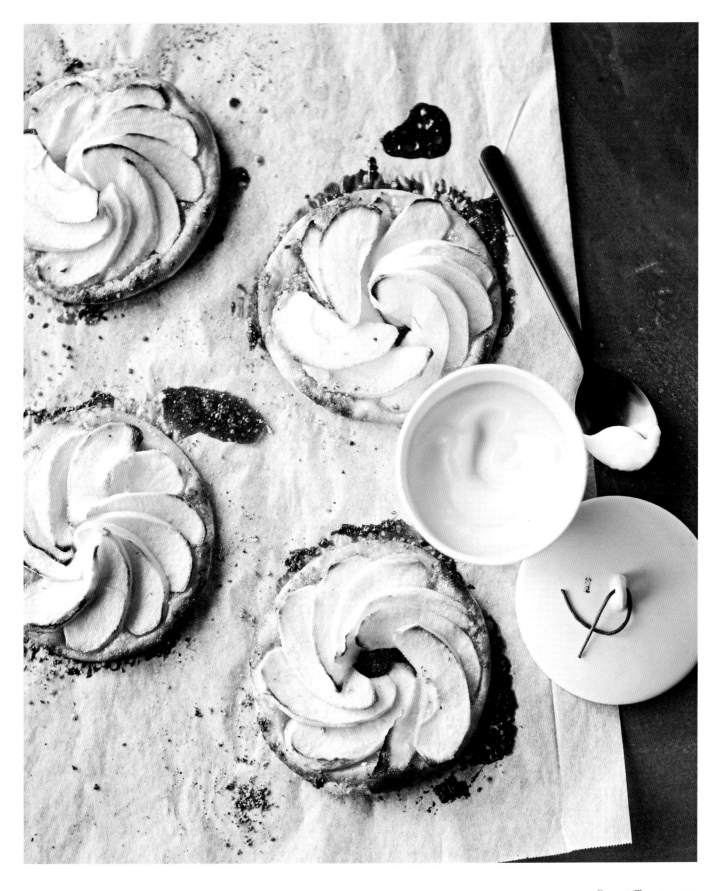

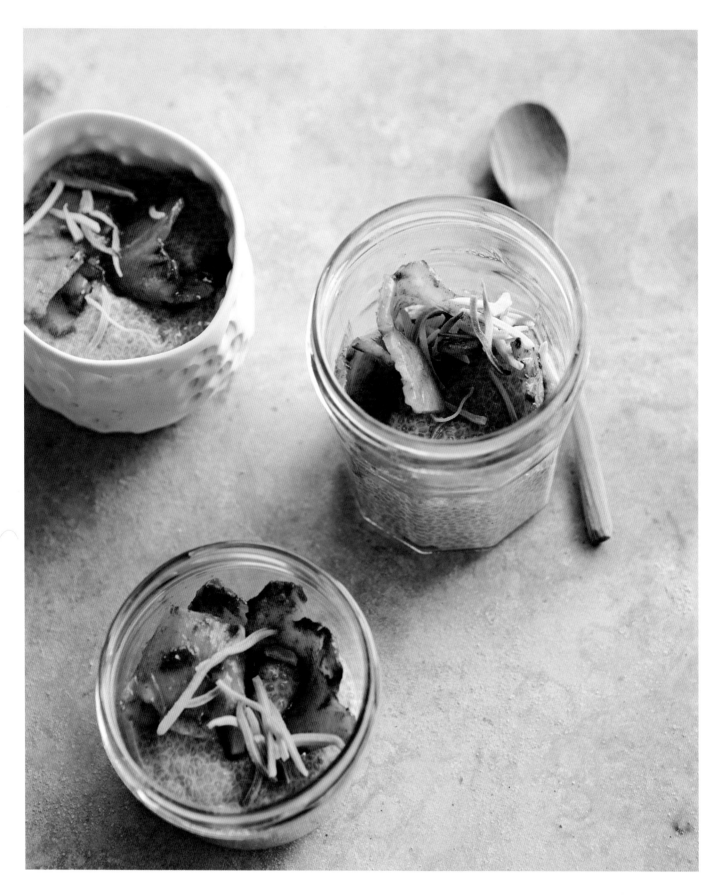

ALMOND CHIA PUDDINGS
with CARAMELISED PINEAPPLE

Chia seeds are a rich source of B vitamins and also contain some calcium, iron and magnesium. When mixed with liquid, the chia seeds take on the consistency of a gel, which can be used to replace eggs in baking recipes.

Ingredients

250 ml (9 fl oz/1 cup) unsweetened almond milk

125 ml (4 fl oz/½ cup) unsweetened coconut water

50 g (1¾ oz/¼ cup) white chia seeds

1 teaspoon ground ginger

1 tablespoon shredded coconut

pinch of ground cinnamon

½ small pineapple, thinly sliced

Method

1 Pour the almond milk and coconut water into a bowl. Add the chia seeds and half the ginger, and stir until combined. Cover and refrigerate for 2–3 hours or until thickened.

2 Heat a small non-stick frying pan over medium heat. Add the shredded coconut and cook, stirring, for 2 minutes or until golden brown. Transfer to a plate and set aside.

3 Reheat the frying pan over high heat. Sprinkle the cinnamon and remaining ginger over the pineapple. Cook for 1–2 minutes on each side or until the pineapple is golden and caramelised. Transfer to a plate to cool.

4 Spoon the almond chia mixture into four glasses. Serve topped with the caramelised pineapple and toasted coconut.

Serves 4

Preparation 10 minutes +

3 hours chilling

Cooking 5 minutes

Nutrition	Per serve
Energy (kJ)	470
Protein (g)	3
Carbohydrate (g)	8
Starches (g)	1
Sugars (g)	7
Exchanges	0.5
Portions	1
GI	Medium
GL	Low
Protein:carbohydrate ratio	0.38
Fat (g)	5
Saturated fat (g)	1
Unsaturated fat (g)	4
Saturated:unsaturated ratio	0.25
Fibre (g)	7
Sodium (mg)	35
Potassium (mg)	210
Sodium:potassium ratio	0.17
Gluten free?	Yes

notes

If you are using fresh coconut, carefully pierce the soft indented eye of the husk with a metal skewer and drain it over a bowl to collect the water. Try other fruits such as caramelised bananas or nectarines.

BAKED CHOCOLATE EGG CUSTARDS

Good-quality dark chocolate that has a cocoa content of 70% or higher
will be rich in antioxidants and will also contain less added sugar than
low-quality brands.

Ingredients

375 ml (13 fl oz/1½ cups)
    reduced-fat milk
50 g (1¾ oz) 70% cocoa
    dark chocolate
1 vanilla bean, split lengthways
1 teaspoon chai masala
    powder
2 eggs, at room temperature
2 teaspoons Natvia sweetener
pinch of freshly grated
    nutmeg
20 raspberries

Method

1 Preheat the oven to 170°C (325°F). Put four 125 ml
(4 fl oz/½ cup) capacity ramekins in a roasting tin.

2 Pour the milk into a small saucepan. Break the
chocolate into small pieces and add to the pan,
along with the vanilla seeds and the chai masala
powder. Cook over medium heat until the mixture
is just below boiling point. Remove the pan from
the heat and set aside to cool for 10 minutes.

3 Use an electric mixer with a whisk attachment
to whisk the eggs and sweetener for 1 minute or
until frothy. Slowly pour the warm milk into the
egg mixture and stir until well combined. Strain
the custard mixture into the prepared dishes
and sprinkle with the nutmeg.

4 Pour enough boiling water into the roasting tin
to reach halfway up the sides of the ramekins and
bake for 35–40 minutes or until the custards are
set but still slightly wobbly.

5 Refrigerate the custards for 2 hours or until cold,
then serve topped with the raspberries.

Serves 4
Preparation 10 minutes +
10 minutes cooling and
2 hours chilling
Cooking 45 minutes

Nutrition	Per serve
Energy (kJ)	650
Protein (g)	8
Carbohydrate (g)	14
Starches (g)	2
Sugars (g)	12
Exchanges	1
Portions	1.5
GI	Low
GL	Low
Protein:carbohydrate ratio	0.57
Fat (g)	8
Saturated fat (g)	4
Unsaturated fat (g)	4
Saturated:unsaturated ratio	1
Fibre (g)	1
Sodium (mg)	90
Potassium (mg)	270
Sodium:potassium ratio	0.33
Gluten free?	Yes

note

*Chai masala powder is a dry Indian spice mix made up of cloves,
ginger, cassia, cardamom and pepper. It can be found in Asian
grocery stores, or you can make your own.*

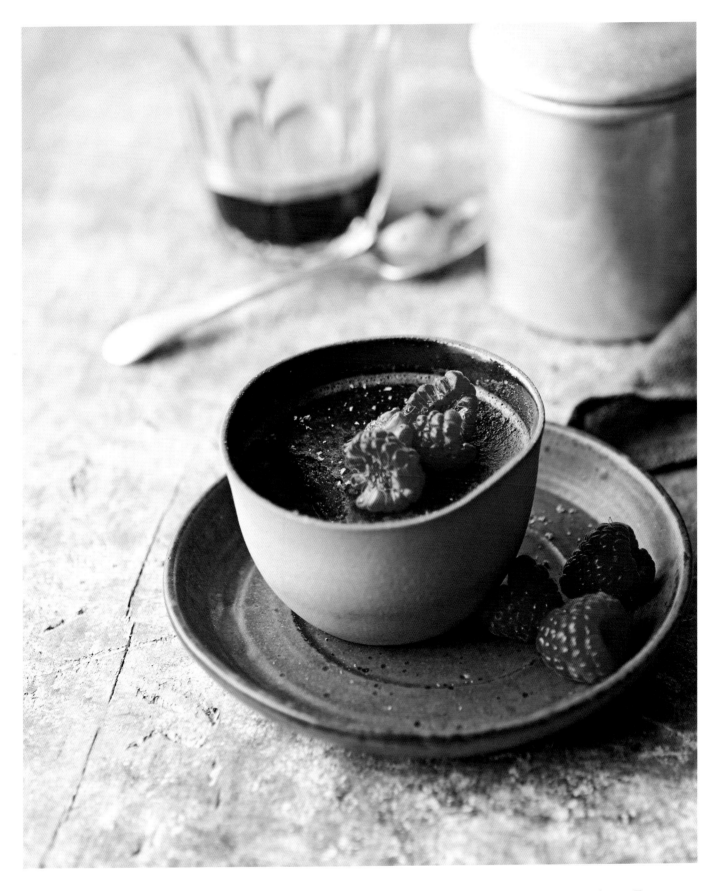

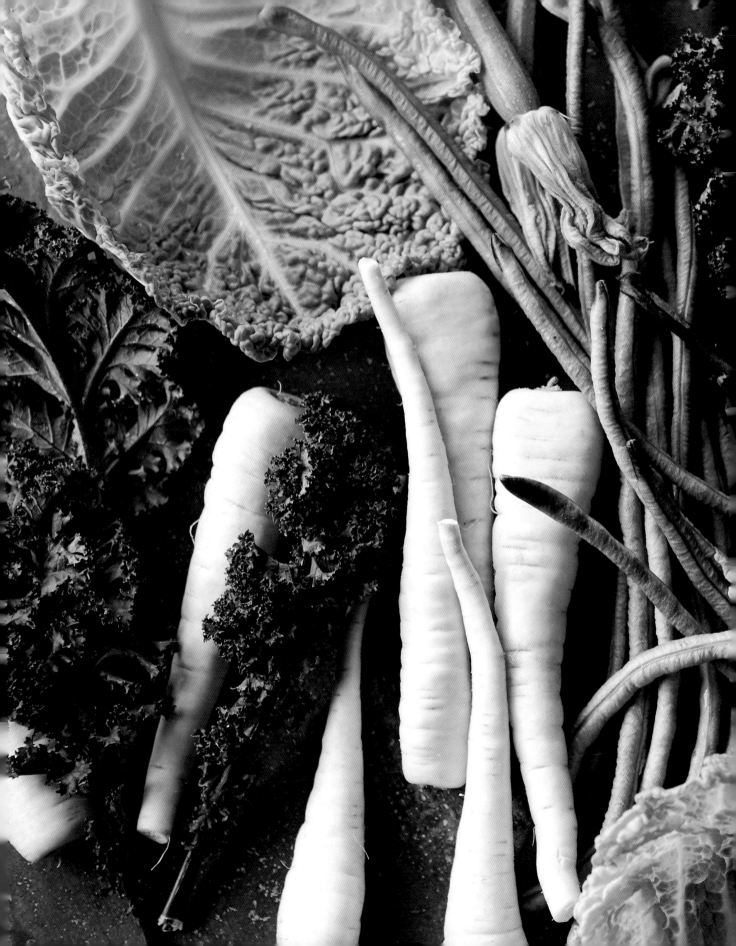

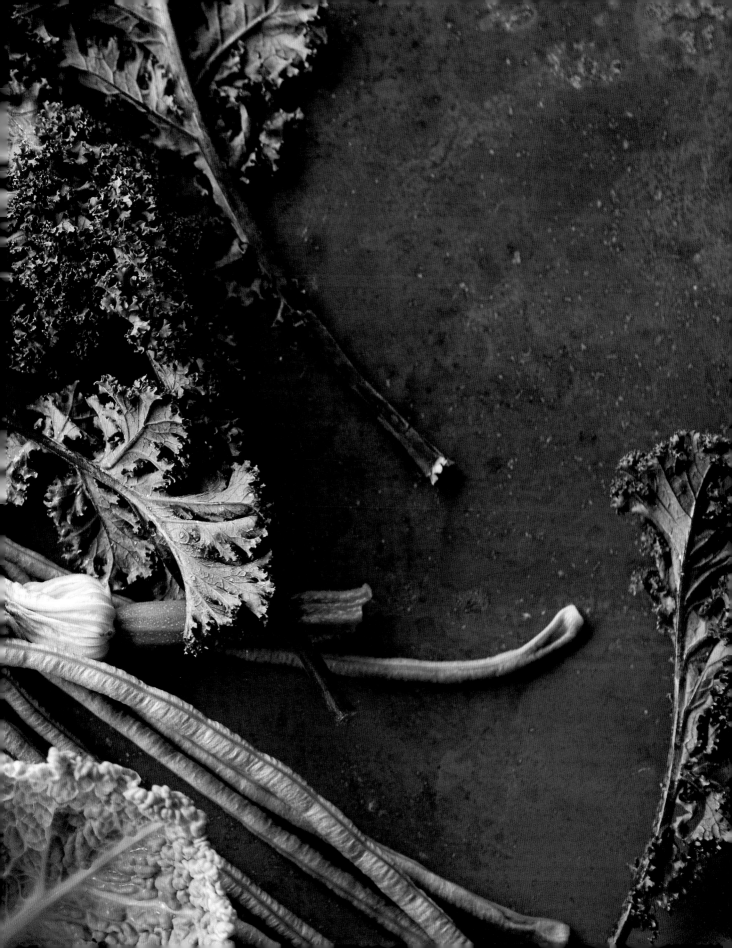

Index

Recipes are printed in *italics*.

A

adenosine triphosphate (ATP) 28

ageing 3, 5, 7

alcohol 15, 50–2

  content in popular drinks 51

  and diabetes 50, 52

  energy density 50

  standard drink 50, 52

  and weight 57–8

allergy 10

Almond chia puddings with caramelised
   pineapple 217

amaranth salad, Brussels sprout, kale
   and 141

American Diabetes Association 17, 26

  management goals 25–6

amino acids 28–9, 30

amylopectin 31

amylose 31

antibodies 10

antioxidants 50

appetite, increased 3, 12

apples

  Apple crumbles 210

  French apple tarts 214

arteries, hardening 50

artificial sweeteners 18–19

  risk of diabetes 18

  and weight 18–19

aspartame 18

atherosclerosis 50

ATP (adenosine triphosphate) 28

avocado 41

  Avocado cream 103

B

Baked chocolate egg custards 218

Baked lemon thyme chicken with sumac pumpkin
   and spinach 179

Balsamic chicken with potato and fennel bake 170

Barbecued corn with avocado cream 103

C

Acknowledgements

My grandfather was the first person I knew who had type 2 diabetes, and as a young child I was scared that one day I might develop it too. He was my first inspiration. My first full-time job was in central New South Wales and it was there that I first met the young woman who was to become my wife. I later found out she had type 1 diabetes. She was my second inspiration. We ended up having two children, and the evidence suggests that both are at increased risk of developing type 1 and type 2 diabetes. They are my third inspiration.

I first started working with people with diabetes during my internship at Royal Perth Hospital, and have never stopped working with them. Diabetes is now such a common condition throughout Australia and the world. The people I have seen over the past twenty years have taught me a lot, and helped me to gain knowledge and wisdom. They have also provided me with inspiration for writing this book.

Along the way I have had the pleasure of working with a range of talented and dedicated colleagues including dietitians, nutritionists, diabetes educators, general practitioners, endocrinologists, exercise physiologists and so on, who have encouraged and inspired me.

I hope this book helps people with pre-diabetes, diabetes and their carers to better understand the condition and to manage it as best they can. I hope some are indeed able to reverse their diabetes.

About the Author

Dr Alan Barclay is an Accredited Practising Dietitian and Nutritionist, and completed a PhD at the University of Sydney in the mid 2000s on the association between glycaemic carbohydrate and the risk of developing lifestyle-related diseases. Alan is currently the Chief Scientific Officer at Glycemic Index Foundation (part-time). He worked for Diabetes Australia as Head of research in both a full-time and part-time capacity from 1998–2014, and has worked in clinical dietetics and has maintained a private practice in Sydney since 1995. Alan is an official Media Spokesperson for the Dietitians Association of Australia and has appeared frequently in newspapers, magazines, radio and television news. He has published more than 30 peer-reviewed articles in the scientific literature and is a co-author of *The New Glucose Revolution: Diabetes & Pre-diabetes Handbook*, *Low GI Diet: Managing Type 2 Diabetes* and *The Ultimate Guide to Sugars & Sweeteners*.

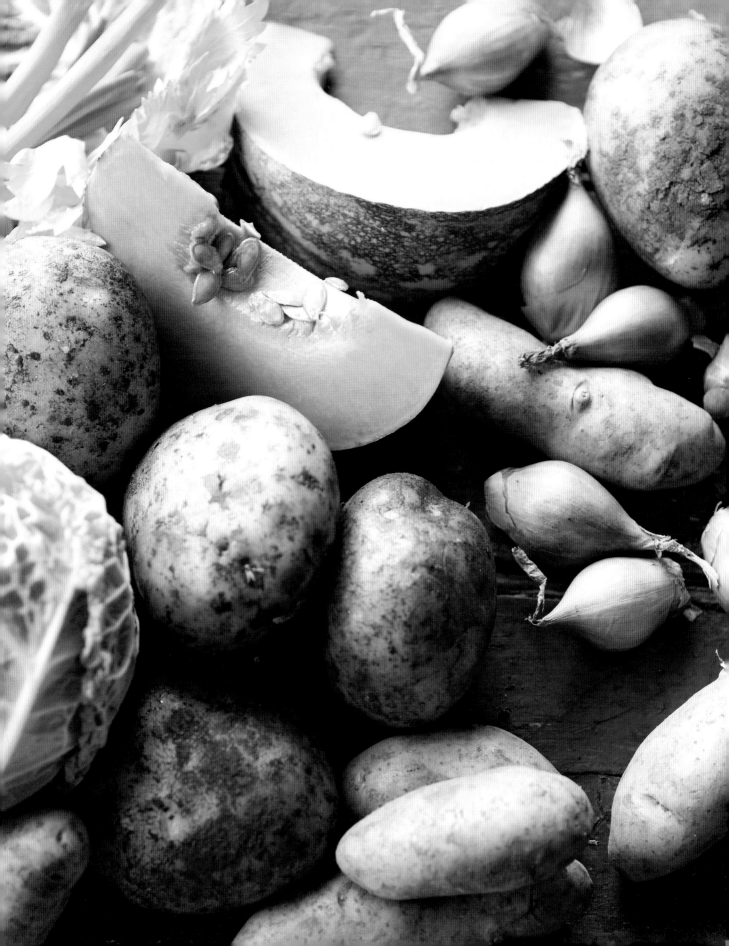

Published in 2016 by Murdoch Books, an imprint of Allen & Unwin

Murdoch Books Australia
83 Alexander Street
Crows Nest NSW 2065
Phone: +61 (0) 2 8425 0100
Fax: +61 (0) 2 9906 2218
murdochbooks.com.au
info@murdochbooks.com.au

Murdoch Books UK
Erico House, 6th Floor
93–99 Upper Richmond Road
Putney, London SW15 2TG
Phone: +44 (0) 20 8785 5995
murdochbooks.co.uk
info@murdochbooks.co.uk

For Corporate Orders & Custom Publishing contact Noel Hammond,
National Business Development Manager, Murdoch Books Australia

Publisher: Jane Morrow
Editorial Manager: Emma Hutchinson
Design Manager: Hugh Ford
Project Editor: Justine Harding
Design: Dan Peterson and Jacqui Porter, Northwood Green
Photographer: Chris Chen
Stylist: Michelle Noerianto
Recipe Development and Home Economist: Theressa Klein
Production Manager: Alex Gonzalez

A cataloguing-in-publication entry is available from the catalogue of the National Library of Australia at
nla.gov.au.

ISBN 978 1 74336 614 1 Australia
ISBN 978 1 74336 631 8 UK.

A catalogue record for this book is available from the British Library.

Colour reproduction by Splitting Image Colour Studio Pty Ltd, Clayton, Victoria
Printed by Hang Tai Printing Company Limited, China

IMPORTANT: Those who might be at risk from the effects of salmonella poisoning (the elderly, pregnant women, young children and those suffering from immune deficiency diseases) should consult their doctor with any concerns about eating raw eggs.

OVEN GUIDE: You may find cooking times vary depending on the oven you are using. For fan-forced ovens, as a general rule, set the oven temperature to 20°C (35°F) lower than indicated in the recipe.

MEASURES GUIDE: We have used 20 ml (4 teaspoon) tablespoon measures. If you are using a 15 ml (3 teaspoon) tablespoon add an extra teaspoon of the ingredient for each tablespoon specified.